Palgrave Texts in Counselling and Psychotherapy

Series Editors
Arlene Vetere
Family Therapy and Systemic Practice
VID Specialized University
Oslo, UK

Rudi Dallos
Clinical Psychology
Plymouth University
Plymouth, UK

This series introduces readers to the theory and practice of counselling and psychotherapy across a wide range of topical issues. Ideal for both trainees and practitioners, the books will appeal to anyone wishing to use counselling and psychotherapeutic skills and will be particularly relevant to workers in health, education, social work and related settings. The books in this series emphasise an integrative orientation weaving together a variety of models including, psychodynamic, attachment, trauma, narrative and systemic ideas. The books are written in an accessible and readable style with a focus on practice. Each text offers theoretical background and guidance for practice, with creative use of clinical examples.

Arlene Vetere, Professor of Family Therapy and Systemic Practice at VID Specialized University, Oslo, Norway.

Rudi Dallos, Emeritus Professor, Dept. of Clinical Psychology, University of Plymouth, UK.

Charley Shults

Attachment Centred Therapy

Therapeutic Practice With Attachment Issues

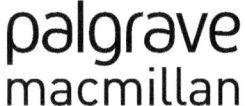

Charley Shults
Attachment Centered Therapy
Manchester, UK

ISSN 2662-9127 ISSN 2662-9135 (electronic)
Palgrave Texts in Counselling and Psychotherapy
ISBN 978-3-031-60850-6 ISBN 978-3-031-60851-3 (eBook)
https://doi.org/10.1007/978-3-031-60851-3

Cover Credit: Sergey Ryumin

This Palgrave Macmillan imprint is published by the registered company Springer Nature Switzerland AG.
The registered company address is: Gewerbestrasse 11, 6330 Cham, Switzerland

If disposing of this product, please recycle the paper.

For lovely
Lou
The love of my life

To Charley: In Memoriam

Dear Reader

Charley died unexpectedly during the last stages of the production of his book. Writing this book meant so much to Charley. It is his first book. Some say we all have one book in us – Charley had plans to write two more! I, Arlene, have known Charley for over 20 years. I, Rudi, have known Charley during his writing of this book and in meetings with training. He was generous in his acknowledgment of our work, and it was a delight to see how we were all pursuing similar interests and future plans.

We both know him to be a wise, modest and compassionate therapist and a gentle, humorous man. As you read his book, his wisdom and experience will shine through every page, and you will come to meet him and know him as we do. We both draw some comfort from knowing that Charley had seen his book in PDF format prior to publication, and in knowing that you will enjoy learning from his long, rich and varied experience.

Arlene Vetere and Rudi Dallos
Series Editors

ACKNOWLEDGEMENTS

There are many people to whom I owe gratitude for this book being published. I have no doubt that there are some who I will inadvertently overlook, for which (like any good A+ strategist) I will apologize in advance! There are many others that I will include in reference to the organizations in which we jointly served. This is intentional due to limitations of time and space and also to provide some degree of cover for the first category! Those that I will name here are the ones who stand out in my mind, both for the length of our association and for the depth of our exploration.

I begin with the most important, the most pervasive, and that is my wife, Louise, or Dr Louise Atkin in her capacity as a child and adolescent psychiatrist and therapist. We met at the IASA (International Association for the Study of Attachment) Conference in Frankfurt, Germany, in September, 2012. Given that she works primarily with children and young adults on attachment issues and I work with adults and couples, it was, one might say, a marriage made in heaven. Together we have explored ideas, techniques, and possibilities with regard to both our personal and professional evolution in attachment. We practice what we preach, if you will forgive another religious allusion. Our life together is the living embodiment of what I am presenting here. More important for the thesis of this book, Louise began to apply the ideas and methods of Attachment Centred Therapy (ACT) with her clients, or patients in the medical setting, and had immediate success, as I did when I first began to explore the concept. She has also been very patient with me (for a C+ strategist!) as I have devoted significant time to getting this book done. It's only taken me 20 years!

Next is Dr Arlene Vetere, my supervisor, my mentor, my friend. Arlene, a highly accomplished practitioner, author, and clinician, encouraged me to submit this book to Palgrave Macmillan for publication in their Palgrave Texts in Counselling and Psychotherapy series. It had never occurred to me to have the temerity to write a book for other professionals to use. Arlene encouraged me to do so, and with her guidance and that of her colleague, who is next in this list, the book has been shepherded into what it is now. Arlene has been my support throughout the process. It was she who first recognized the resemblance of Attachment Narrative Therapy (ANT) to Attachment Centred Therapy.

My intent initially was to write a book that might be of interest to anyone, both therapists, their clients, and do-it-yourselfers who wanted guidance in their own journey of recovery. It also addressed a number of societal issues, including cosmology. It was Arlene who suggested that I pare it down to a focused book for therapists. I am glad she did.

Her co-author and co-creator of ANT, Dr Rudi Dallos, then took over the task of actually editing the book into the final version to be submitted to Palgrave Macmillan. Rudi has been a good editor. He has advised, questioned, and cajoled me into making changes that make the book more succinct, more evidence based, more directly relevant to the subject that it purports to treat. I can feel his excitement at interacting with two approaches, ANT and ACT, that have so much in common. To have two such accomplished scholars and clinicians assisting me has been a great blessing. I am very thankful for their generosity and giving spirit.

Of course, as you have discovered in reading this book, Dr Paticia Crittenden and the Dynamic Maturational Model of Attachment (DMM) plays a leading role. It was Pat who recommended Arlene when I was looking for a supervisor knowledgeable about attachment. It was Pat who explained to me the difference between the mainstream model of attachment in the USA, the Berkeley or ABC+D model, and the DMM, and why the research articles I was reading were not lending clarity to my understanding of attachment, but rather confusion, because it did not make sense. It was her elucidation of the DMM that has led me to my understanding of attachment today. And if I've got any of it wrong, then that is my error, not hers. I am amazed at what she has done. It is tempting to say 'single-handedly,' but that is not quite right. She has had many colleagues along the way who have helped her in developing and promoting her model. Many of them have been important to me in my development as well. Andrea Landini is her primary collaborator. He is the co-author of their book, *Assessing Adult Attachment*,[1] and was her co-trainer as well in our training course. There are many others, of course. And this is where I restrain myself, because if I name one, or a few, I will miss out others.

Pat had the courage to break out on her own. To look at new data with new eyes. To actualize her belief that in the discrepancies lies the new learning. It is this spirit of intellectual enquiry that has led to her expansion of the original Ainsworth categories into the current DMM model. She has indeed been true to the vision of Bowlby and Ainsworth that their model would be 'refined and extended,' to use their words. She has had the courage to endure shunning by her peers in the attachment establishment because she could not agree that it was safety that organized attachment, that the best we could do with new patterns of attachment was to label them 'disorganized,' or that attachment was 'transmitted' from mother to child in some mysterious way. Although I was not present in those early days, I was early enough to be a founding member of the International Association for the Study of Attachment in 2007.

I also have great gratitude for another mentor, teacher and colleague, Dr Patrick Carnes. I met Pat Carnes at a South-Eastern Conference on Alcohol and Drugs in Atlanta, Georgia. We had a long association before I came to the UK. I was active in the International Institute of Trauma and Addiction Professionals and the National Council on Sexual Addiction and Compulsivity (now the Society for the Advancement of Sexual Health) and served on the boards of both those organizations. It was my years of service on those boards and the commensurate rewards that led me to assiduously resist the temptations to serve on the IASA board!

Pat Carnes, like Pat Crittenden, has written many books, trained many therapists, and broken new ground in their fields. I have found it very exciting to be in on the cutting edge of development in both the addiction and trauma and the attachment field. It was with Pat Carnes that I first discussed my ideas regarding addiction, attachment, and trauma, that are presented in this book.

Special thanks, too, to my very first supervisors, Robbin McInturff and Jim Cotton at Adult and Child Development Professionals in Birmingham, Alabama. Robbin was my official supervisor and Jim was an unofficial supervisor. During that time Robbin was voted Supervisor of the Year by the American Counselling Association. I had nothing to do with her winning that honor. Again, I feel deeply fortunate to have had such an accomplished supervisor, colleague, and mentor. Another supervisor from that period was Dr Don Brown. I was a member of Don's systemic family therapists supervision group until I left to come to England.

I also want to acknowledge the contribution of my late wife, Dr Nanci Turner-Shults. She had achieved her dream of becoming a professor at the University of Alabama when she was tragically struck with illness that quickly led to her death. It was she who suggested to me that I become a counsellor. She stood by me during my active addiction disorder and into recovery. She helped me get my start in counselling with my first job at the treatment centre. She introduced me to the idea of Bowlby's attachment theory, and the rudimentary A, B and C attachment strategies.

There are many others, of course, and when I think of the many friends, colleagues and teachers over the years, I smile with gladness. So please forgive me for not naming you all.

I also want to thank my parents. They did the best they could, and in many ways it was a piss-poor job. That's the truth. But they had to struggle with their own demons: their own abuse, their own addictions, their own shame. And even though they were not always impeccable with their word, they gave me a commitment to some kind of integrity, where one must account to oneself for ones actions in life. They instilled an ethic of being kind to others, of looking down on no one, because there but for circumstance go I, and of being unimpressed by material wealth because there but for circumstance go any of us. Whatever else, they helped me to realize that our circumstances in life determine who we are, what we believe, and how we treat others. And most of all, in the realm of trauma and addiction, they gave me a lot of good material to work with!

Saving the best for last, I am deeply grateful to my clients whose stories they have allowed me to share with you. Their courage, their commitment, their dedication to making their lives and the lives of others better has been steadfast. To trust me to share their journey with them has been an honour. And remember,

It takes courage to grow up
And become
Who you really are
  e.e. Cummings

NOTE

1. Crittenden, P. M., & Landini, A. (2011). *Assessing adult attachment: A dynamic-maturational approach to discourse analysis.* WW Norton & Company.

CONTENTS

CHAPTER 1

Attachment Centred Therapy

'In the foundling home the child becomes sad and many of them die from sadness'. A Spanish bishop, 1760. Quoted by Robert Karen, *Becoming Attached*[1]

> 'When I wake up in the morning,' she said, 'I am filled with dread.'
> 'Really?' I replied. 'And what do you think when you feel that?' I asked.
> 'I think, 'What disaster am I going to have to deal with today?"
> 'Oh dear,' I said. 'And what kind of disasters have you ever had to deal with?'
> She thought a moment.
> 'None,' she replied.

I already knew the answer to that question because Andrea and I had been working with her Adult Attachment Interview (AAI) for some time, and I was familiar with her life growing up and as an adult. I also understood why she had that dreadful feeling on awakening. It was her default state: the condition in which one finds oneself when there is nothing to alter the mood one way or another. It was the pathway down which she automatically travelled without stopping to consider whether or not there was something dreadful to deal with.

When you are running for your life, it's hard to stop and think.

C. Shults, *Attachment Centred Therapy*, Palgrave Texts in Counselling and Psychotherapy, https://doi.org/10.1007/978-3-031-60851-3_1

ATTACHMENT CENTRED THERAPY: A HUMANISTIC, INTEGRATIVE THERAPY MODEL

Attachment Centred Therapy (ACT) is an integrative therapy, meaning that it utilizes many—indeed, any—techniques that are useful in correcting what I call 'errors of information processing,' or 'transformations of information,' as Crittenden and Landini call them.[2] They identify these as: (1) erroneous (vs. true); (2) distorted (over or under-emphasized); (3) omitted information; (4) false information (e.g. to mislead); (5) denied information (e.g. to avoid responsibility for causation or to avoid painful recall); (6) delusional information (i.e. false information to resolve discrepancies). While these are not all 'errors' in that some are done intentionally, they are all contrary to 'true' in that they contain some degree of incorrectness.

While we could use 'information processing that we can change that will lead to a more coherent narrative and presumably a better life for oneself and others,' that is cumbersome. We could also call them transformations of information, the term used in Crittenden and Landini's book. But that term, too, includes transformations that are accurate and helpful. We will identify these 'errors' by discourse markers, a term of art that allows us to analyse the coherence of the clients narrative of their lives and then, by a sort of reverse engineering, create a more coherent narrative.

It is also worth recognizing at the outset that the term 'discourse markers' will be used both generically to include virtually anything that helps us to identify the aforementioned 'errors' but also specific discourse markers. We will look at these in some detail as we go along. However, the purpose of this book is not to train you in discourse analysis. It is rather to introduce you to the specific form of therapy that I have evolved over some decades for working with clients once you get the information as to their attachment strategies and any unresolved trauma, abuse or neglect, and grief associated with that. I hope it will also help to discern more information from your interactions with your clients, and your knowledge of their interactions with others, whether you know how to code a transcript or not.

These errors, distortions, or transformations of information (I will use the terms synonymously) may be conscious or unconscious. We will see a fairly vivid example of a conscious omission early on with 'the long kiss goodnight.' Other ways are unconscious. They operate automatically at the unconscious mind level to produce an emotional response without the conscious mind's awareness of what is happening. Typically, the A strategy filters out negative emotional information and the facts that go with it, and the C strategy filters out cognitive information that is contrary to their feelings. The B strategy uses accurate cognitive and emotional information. These errors can be identified using assessment instruments, with the focus being on the Adult Attachment Interview. My wife, a child and adolescent psychiatrist, also uses ACT using the Transition to Adulthood Attachment Interview (TAAI), and I sometimes use it as well when working with teens. With experience and practice, we can identify them real time, in spoken or written language, when working with our clients. With effective interventions, clients can begin to recognize when they are distorting information and correct it, also in the here and now. This learning is then input into the information processing, resulting in new and better outcomes, making this an iterative or recursive process.

I first heard of attachment theory in about 2000. An appropriate time: the turn of the millennium. My ex-wife who was working on her Ph.D. in Counselling at the University of Alabama told me about it. She told me about the three basic strategies of A, B, and C, and how those three strategies affect behaviour via our information processing. Basically, the A strategy, sometimes called 'avoidant,' relies on cognition excessively and avoids negative feelings. They get satisfaction by pleasing others, especially attachment figures. The B strategy we can call 'balanced,' meaning that they use a balance of both cognitive and affective information to meet needs and please themselves and others by being sensitive and responsive to the needs of both. The C strategy I choose to call 'coercive,' meaning they use negative feelings in order to justify themselves and motivate others to meet their needs. They disregard cognitive information that is in conflict with their emotional conclusions.

The information was intriguing to me, and I thought it might be the missing link that I had been looking for to answer a couple of fundamental questions.

The first question was highly relevant for my professional life. As a counsellor in an addiction treatment centre and then as a private practitioner, I had often wondered why people who knew they had a life-threatening illness that, in recovery parlance, was going to rob you before it killed you, would continue to do that behaviour even though they had been given a tried-and-true method of recovery? Better yet, why did they, after many years of recovery and experiencing 'a new freedom and a new happiness,'[3] (a) relapse, (b) take up another addiction, or (c) go home one night and put a bullet through their brain? It didn't make sense to me. Something was missing.

The second question was very personal. Why couldn't my wife and I, both professional counsellors, resolve the conflict in our relationship and live happily ever after? Or at least, more often than not? I had found Notarius and Markman's highly effective book, *We Can Work It Out*,[4] and I was using it successfully with many of my clients. The techniques were sound. They worked with many, but not all my clients. Better yet, why did I find myself in sessions thinking, 'Gee, I wish my wife and I could do what you guys just did!' Again, something was missing.

I thought that attachment theory might be the missing piece. I hypothesized that the information we needed was buried in the unconscious mind. I had been using NLP (Neurolinguistic Programming)[5] for many years before getting into counselling. NLP posits that our behaviour is based on programmes that are embedded neurologically and linguistically in the unconscious mind. The way to change behaviour, then, is to change the programmes that run the behaviour. (But, for the behaviourists among us, remember that, like clockwork, it works the other way round, too. It just might take longer.) For those therapists who consider NLP to be beneath them, may I refer you to books of a more noble pedigree, by Daniel Kahneman[6] and John Bargh.[7] In the latter book, there is an interesting vignette that illustrates the point when Bargh relates a dream that was key to resolving the dilemma that had his conscious, rational, mind stumped!

Perhaps, since attachment theory dealt with those earliest days of life, that would hold the key to resolving these questions. Since conscious memory formation doesn't begin until later in life, those early events and the memory of them would be imbedded in the neurology of the unconscious mind. We would have no conscious memory of them. As my Aunt Lillian used to say when something awful happened to a young child, 'Oh don't worry. *It* won't remember it when *it* grows up.' She was right, of course, about the *conscious* mind not being able to recall the event. But she was wrong because the *unconscious* mind will retain the information in the form of an implicit memory.[8]

I read Robert Karen's book, *Becoming Attached*,[9] and I began to read the research literature of attachment. I began to tentatively explain the theory to my clients and why I thought that it might apply to them. At that time, my work was predominantly with addictive disorders, trauma, abuse and neglect, and the family dynamics that accompanied these problems. My hypothesis was that these problems were rooted in family dynamics, deeply buried in the unconscious mind. I got immediate results.

One client, when I had discussed this with him, responded, 'Oh, you mean I've become attached to my drug of choice instead of to a person?' I hadn't meant that at all! But, we learn from our clients. I realized immediately that he was right: he *had* become attached to his drug. It had become his source of nurturing, of comfort, and that had become the source of his feelings of self-worth, safety and security, and higher needs as well. The fear of losing that comfort, that refuge, is what makes giving up so hard.

But carrying on till death? Why? Seeking comfort was one thing, but the comfort of death is another entirely. And then I got the answer.

My phone rang. It was our secretary. 'Turn on your tv,' she said. 'Why?' 'Just turn it on.' 'Which channel?' 'It doesn't matter. Just turn it on.' I did. I was having trouble making sense of what I was seeing. What was going on? The tv commentators were equally baffled. After a few moments, the second plane appeared and flew straight into the south tower. Well, that answered one important question. The first one wasn't an accident, either. We all saw what happened that day. But as I watched, a strange thing started happening, as if things were not strange enough already.

Objects were falling from the building. At some point it dawned on me: those are people. They continued to fall until the towers fell. And then the other realization dawned. That is why people will sacrifice themselves, when it is bad enough, to escape pain, uncertainty. Yet those people *knew* what was about to happen to them. So they could make a conscious choice as to whether to stay and endure the fear and anguish, or whether to end it quickly by jumping. I related that to how addictive behaviours can be persistent, whether consciously or unconsciously choosing to avoid the pain of withdrawal and the fear of having to cope without the addictive behaviour. As one veteran put it, when I worked as a veterans services officer, 'I just want to turn off my mind.'

I was also able to see a marked contrast between those who suffered from PTSD (post-traumatic stress disorder) and those who didn't, even though both groups had been exposed to the trauma of war. Why did some suffer from PTSD while others got past the trauma and went on to resume life unimpeded? Was this attachment related too? The answer, I believe, lies in the field of research that inspired Bowlby's original work[10]: ethology. And to understand that, we need to turn to the work of René Spitz.[11]

Children who had been institutionalized were dying in great numbers in the early decades of the twentieth century. Their physical needs were being met, including medical care, and there were no explanations within the understanding of medicine and child care to explain it.[12] What made it even worse was that the germ theory of disease had caught on by then, and so the institutions' administrators doubled down on isolating these children in the belief that it was some pathogen that was causing their deaths.

What Spitz concluded was that it was *the lack of an attachment figure* that was causing these deaths. Three phases that children went through when they were separated from their caregivers were identified: protest, despair, and detachment. It would be during the despair phase, I imagine, that they would die. One may see this process in a video, *John,* made by the Robertsons.[13] In other words, these children were dying of grief from the lack of attachment.

Attachment is what keeps us alive. Without attachment, we die. With insecure attachment, we fear death, and sometimes we actually do die.

And if there was any remaining doubt, we have another unfortunate and inadvertent sociological experiment: Ceausescu's Romanian orphans.[14]

Porges' polyvagal theory[15] gives us possible mechanisms for these deaths, and the concept of vagal tone helps to explain the default state to which we return when there is nothing to keep us from it. Dawkins[16] hypothesizes an extinction or death gene. His theory, because genes are interested only in their own survival, *in the species,* is that to have a gene that responds when an *individual* is not receiving sufficient nurturing to survive and then decides to extinguish that individual so that other off-spring with the same genetic inheritance will have an improved chance of survival and thus preserve that genetic heritage, is evolutionarily sound.

But the point is, whatever the theory to explain it, these children died in huge numbers when they had no attachment figure, as the Spanish Bishop quoted by Karen and reproduced at the beginning of this chapter had observed.

ATTACHMENT TRAUMA

I continue to be puzzled when I hear professionals talk about having a traumatized client but not being able to find a traumatic event to which to relate it. Attachment trauma is the original trauma in my opinion. Our survival, over millions of years of evolution to become *homo sapiens,* depended on our caregivers being there for us. The equation is simple, and still in play. It works like this:

1. Mammals require more parental care than other species.
2. Primates require more parental care than other mammals.
3. *Homo sapiens* require more parental car than other primates.
4. Offspring who get this parental care in the optimal amount for their environment are more likely to survive than those who don't.
5. Any genetic behavioural propensities that lead to the establishment of a protective relationship are enhanced by survival and reproduction.
6. Any genetic behavioural propensities that lead to the diminishment of a protective relationship are extinguished by a failure of survival and reproduction.
7. The failure of protective relating can, in some instances, itself lead to failure to survive.
8. Sequalae of a failure of protection include diminished reproductive capacity, diminished ability to thrive, for example lower weight, lower intelligence, increased illnesses, etc.
9. Extreme emotions of terror at the lack of parental protection are experienced and encoded traumatically and endure via enhancement of neurological pathways.
10. The only way offspring can know that they are safe from death is by close, rewarding contact with their parents.

In other words, the lack of being held and comforted by your caregiver results in a neurological message in the mind, 'Oh shit! I'm gonna die now!' This is the basis of attachment trauma. It's not what *happens,* it is what *doesn't happen.* Of course, this does not mean that there are no instances where infants and young children are traumatized by something happening to them. Sometimes there are circumstances in which parents kill their children. There are many instances of trauma, abuse, and neglect. Sometimes it goes on for years. And it is more likely that parents who are neglectful or abusive to their children in early childhood will be more likely to neglect or abuse as they mature. Nor do I deny that there are children who have secure attachments that are then disrupted by one of the ACEs (adverse childhood experiences): death; divorce; serious mental illness; trauma, abuse and neglect, other losses; and poverty.

My clients typically have PTSD symptoms, and yet there is no recognizable trauma in their background. Often they have difficulty remembering their early childhood experiences.

Attachment Centred Therapy places attachment at the centre for the above reasons. It is the missing link needed to explain and deal with dysfunctional behaviours and both interpersonal and internal conflict. Because these responses are programmed into the unconscious mind, the aim of ACT is to reprogramme the unconscious mind, since that is where the initial information processing is accomplished and the outcome is presented to our conscious mind for disposition based on our representation of it to ourselves. We use 'perceptual filters' to let through some information, to exclude other information, and to distort or colour other information. No information gets through without passing through these perceptual filters. Our goal is to identify where there are errors being introduced into perceptual filtering and to correct it.

VALIDITY OF ACT

ACT is a method of correcting the errors of information processing inherent in A and C and developing the processing needed for B. I feel confident in asserting that ACT is a new approach to psychotherapy with high validity. As such, I am proposing that ACT is a scientifically valid approach to psychotherapy, meaning that with accurate observation we can use the theory to make predictions that are then borne out by the results. I have three sources of information on which I base this.

Observation

First is observation. All good science is based on observation. Just as the Dynamic Maturational Model (DMM) is based on observation, so is ACT. My training prior to therapy had been as an artillery officer and gunnery instructor in the U.S. Army where we literally learned to observe, report data, and calculate corrections, and as a lawyer where we learned to gather the facts, develop a theory to explain the facts, and seek a remedy based on the theory. Obviously both factually oriented enterprises that worked well with my bias towards cognition in information processing. However, neglecting my negative emotions and the consequences of unmet needs meant growing frustration and shame, resulting in treatment, recovery, and carrying on to become a therapist. I am therefore highly motivated to help others through my experience.

In applying ACT with my clients, in the early days, I observed positive results in a relatively short period. Three clients, all young females dealing with relationship issues, made rapid progress far more quickly than I had been accustomed to seeing. This pattern has continued, but it is not the only pattern that I see. In some cases, ACT leads to extensive work at a very deep level. The length of time that therapy takes depends on a number of variables. Age is the most obvious, as the older we are the longer new learning takes. Others are support networks, severity of trauma, abuse and neglect or ACEs, and resources for recovery. As a result of these factors, some clients stay in therapy longer, not because they are not making progress but because they are. This is the case with Andrea, with whom we began.

The evidence I offer in this book will be practice-based research which is supported by case detailed and multiple case presentations. This has a rich history in the development of the psychotherapies and arguably offers us more as clinicians than randomized control trials (RCTs), which often tell us very little about the process of therapy and understanding of what works, doesn't work, and why.

Replication: Attachment Narrative Therapy

One way of establishing validity is by replicability. And the best form of replicability, I believe, is when replications occur independently from one another. This replication comes from Attachment Narrative Therapy (ANT).[17,18] Dr. Arlene Vetere is my supervisor, and we have worked together for many years now. She and Dr. Rudi Dallos have developed Attachment Narrative Therapy (ANT), which is a close cousin to ACT. I think the main distinction between them is the theoretical starting place. ANT starts with the family system and then works inwards to the individual. ACT starts with the individual and works outwards towards the family. Really, both approaches do both. For example, in *Systemic Therapy and Attachment Narratives,* the book opens with the story of Alice who came to Drs Dallos and Vetere for help with her autistic son. I have opened this book with the story of Andrea who came to me for help with her anorexic daughter, her difficult marriage, and her family or origin issues.

Attachment Centred Therapy is very similar to Attachment Narrative Therapy.[19] Both use the Dynamic Maturational Model of Attachment in assessing clients and their attachment relationships and strategies. Both believe in the efficacy of systemic approaches: a client and their problems cannot be properly understood without understanding the environment in which they operate. Both recognize that change is rarely about the individual alone. The system in which the person operates will also have to change. Conversely, when one part of a system changes, the rest of the system also changes. ACT was born out of a union between the DMM-AAI and Humanistic/Integrative Psychotherapy. Attachment Narrative Therapy was born out of a union of the DMM-AAI and Systemic Family Therapy.

It seemed evident working in the treatment centre that the family system was fundamental to the development of virtually all addictive disorders. Evidence for this was provided by the observation that patients whose families were supportive of therapy were much more likely to be successful in their recovery than those whose families weren't.

The authors have this to say about ANT:

> Our starting point is the view that the stories we create about our lives are a key component in how we live and how we develop problems and difficulties in our relationships. We create narratives about what has happened to us in our lives and these help shape how we think of our past and importantly how we view and embark on the future. The ANT approach focuses on an important set of stories that we develop about our connections, namely our emotional and sexually intimate relationships, our attachments with others, such as our parents and children, and our dependencies, experiences and expectations of trust in our relationships. Attachment theory emphasises that we have a fundamental need, which appears to be based on an evolutionary survival instinct, to engage in intimate relationships fuelled by this need, starting in infancy, to seek safety and protection with our parents/carers when faced with threats of danger, loss and adversity. These early interactions between the parent and the child produce the experiences that form the material of our developing narratives about ourselves and others. These experiences subsequently come to be shaped into broader narratives and sets of expectations that we generalise to other relationships outside our families. However, narratives are not a passive recording of the past but constitute an active process of continual construction, reconstruction and review. We tell our stories to others and their questions, reactions, comments, additions, revisions and corrections serve to reshape our stories with each telling. As we tell our stories, powerful feelings are evoked, even when we muse to ourselves, which shape how and when we tell our stories—for example: who we tell, what we leave out, forget or defend ourselves from remembering, alter, adjust and edit—and, of course, why we tell. We may also alter our stories according to whom we are telling and thus how safe we feel to be honest, straightforward, open and able to access our memories. Our framework approach therefore shares much with the narrative therapies

in our emphasis on working with people's narratives and relationships to foster change, liberation and release from their interpersonal problems. However, we add an emphasis on the emotional content of people's stories, and as yet unstoried experiences, such as trauma, and in particular on how they manage their feelings and attachments, for example, how they comfort themselves and others in times of anxiety, distress and difficulties. We are particularly interested in how children learn to narrate their experiences and what assists them in developing the skills for open, consistent and coherent communication of their emotional experiences. In addition, we focus on the process of the telling of the narratives to consider what types of self-protective strategies or defences people are employing as painful, shameful, uncomfortable and anxiety-provoking memories are evoked in the telling. This shares some similarities with psychodynamic models in recognising the need to elicit both what is explicit and also what is implicit—what we find harder to articulate, and that which may not yet have reached conscious awareness. This does not involve adopting an 'expert' position of knowing better than the families we see but of finding ways to help them to articulate the more hidden, subjugated and feared aspects of their emotional experiences in their relationships and the self-protective strategies that they may have been employing. Central to this is the creation of a context of safety and trust for families that can help such material to be accessed, illuminated, expanded, expressed and processed.

Dallos, Rudi; Vetere, Arlene. *Systemic Therapy and Attachment Narratives* (pp. 11–12). Taylor and Francis. Kindle Edition.[20] *Used with permission of Rudi Dallos*

Outcome

Successful outcome is the third criterion. Insight alone into the nature of problems does not bring about change unless coupled with action. ACT is a way of combining insight with skill development, primarily by identifying the errors of information processing and correcting them. This ought to lead to improved outcomes for clients. Those outcomes may be subjective based on the client's evaluation of their experience, or objective, to the extent possible, based on the specific criteria of observation by the therapist.

The subjective observations by clients are also confirmed by objective outcomes. The three young women to whom I referred earlier were successful by their criteria by: (1) establishing a caring and committed long-term relationship within 6 months of starting ACT; (2) ending an abusive relationship and having new criteria for their future relationships within

3 months of starting ACT; (3) ending an abusive and exploitive relationship and beginning a satisfying relationship approximately 2.5 years after starting ACT. Another example is a client who, despite being retirement age, made rapid progress and in 6 months was finished. The variables there were: (1) he had been engaged in work on his issues for years, perhaps decades; (2) he was a helping professional with extensive knowledge of how our thoughts and feelings affect us; (3) he had been using dream analysis to probe his unconscious mind content for decades.

This is not to imply that change always comes quickly. The older one is, the longer it takes. The psychosocial circumstances will vary: for example marital status, family support, children, friendships, etc. Many of the clients whose stories I will tell later on in this book I have been working with for many years. They have faithfully come to therapy, not because it isn't effective, but rather, because it is. Their lives and functioning in their relationships have markedly improved over those years. I have selected them for presentation here *because* they have been difficult cases.

Other indicators of outcome: (1) observed instances of changes in information processing within therapy sessions; (2) specific applications of ACT techniques to good effect in their lives; (3) global and deep improvements in information processing that manifest by them making changes in areas of life that either we have not discussed at all or that were only mentioned in passing. This last one was the most surprising to me. Yet, it is an example of the importance of being able to give a coherent narrative of one's life. It also is the predicted outcome of reprogramming the mind to create more balanced and undistorted information processing.

Application

You may or may not be familiar with attachment principles and ideas. Attachment, like mindfulness, is a word that can be incorporated with or without much understanding of what it means or how it works. To paraphrase Eisenhower, the correct application of a principle of knowledge is more important than the mere awareness of its existence. Yet the awareness of its existence is the beginning of enquiry in a desire to know more. I hope this book will give you the courage and the inspiration to begin to apply these techniques and the Attachment Centred Therapy approach with your clients.

My wife, Dr. Louise Atkin, a child and adolescent psychiatrist, has been using ACT with some of her clients for some years now, with good results.

I hope that I am presenting this material in such a way that it will be of assistance to you at whatever level you are practising. And if you want additional help with applying these principles and techniques, please get in touch. I will be happy to help if I can.

THE CORE BELIEFS: A MODEL FOR HOW WE MEET OUR NEEDS AND OTHERS'

Our core beliefs are formed in the earliest days of life and continue to develop as we develop. I learned about core beliefs from Dr. Patrick Carnes, author of *Out of the Shadows*[21] and many other books related to sexually compulsive behaviour and trauma.[22] It was my pleasure to work with Dr. Carnes as a part of IITAP, the International Institute for Trauma and Addiction Professionals, some years ago.

Our core beliefs are held in the deepest part of our being. These beliefs determine: (1) how we feel about ourselves; (2) how we relate to those closest to us; (3) our model of the world; (4) how we meet our needs and the needs of others.

For clients who are struggling with insecure attachment and its effects, these core beliefs may be expressed as: (1) I am a bad, unworthy person (the essence of shame); (2) if you know the *real* me, you won't like me, approve of me, accept me, therefore I have to present a false self to you; (3) the world is not one where I can depend on others to help me meet my needs, therefore I must control, coerce, or be subservient to others; (4) I nurture myself and others by emphasizing my needs and feelings above all else and being preoccupied with our relationship and my fears of abandonment (the C strategy) or emphasizing the needs and feelings of others above all else until I identify them with me, and denying my own needs and feelings and theirs too (the A strategy).

A goal of ACT is to change these core beliefs into: (1) I am a good and worthy person; (2) if you know the real me, you will accept me as I am; (3) I can cooperate with others to meet my and their needs; (4) I nurture myself and others through love, service, and attachment. These are the functional core beliefs that underlie secure attachment.

Each of these aspects can have more elaboration, and of course, most of us will be on a spectrum between the totally dysfunctional beliefs, or attachment insecurity, and the totally functional beliefs, or attachment security. These core beliefs usually lie deeply rooted in our unconscious mind, and so the first step is to bring them into awareness.

Shame-based people do shameful things. We sometimes refer to such people as 'shameless,' but I believe that is wrong. They are so immersed in shame that they don't notice the difference when they do shameful things. That is why it is so easy for some to lie. A's feel their shame deeply, C's project their shame onto others.

To restate the core beliefs: the first core belief about ourselves reflects our beliefs and feelings about whether or not we deserve to get our needs met. The second core belief reflects to what extent we can expose our real selves, our needs and feelings, to others, and particularly to our attachment figures. The third core belief reflects our model of how the world works and is the basis for the prediction of outcomes. The fourth core belief is then about the strategies and tactics that we use to meet our own needs and the needs of others. The result is then fed into the first core belief in a recursive manner.

If we hypothesize that attachment theory gives us a way to understand the strategies for meeting needs, then we also need a model for identifying what those needs are. For that, we turn to a model that has been around for thousands of years but was recently re-discovered and articulated from a more modern, psychological perspective: Maslow's Modified Hierarchy.

NOTES

1. Karen, R. (1998). *Becoming attached: First relationships and how they shape our capacity to love.* Oxford University Press, USA.
2. Crittenden, P. M., & Landini, A. (2011). *Assessing adult attachment: A dynamic-maturational approach to discourse analysis.* WW Norton & Company.
3. Bill, W., & Dick, B. (2011). *Alcoholics Anonymous: the original 1939 edition.* Courier Corporation.
4. Notarius, C., & Markman, H. (1993). *We can work it out: Making sense of marital conflict.* Putnam Adult.
5. Bandler, R., & Grinder, J. (1977). *frogs into PRINCES. Red.* Grinder, J., & Bandler, R. (1981). *Trance-formations.* Moab, UT: Real People Press. Bandler, R., & Grinder, J. (1975). *The structure of magic* (Vol. 1). Palo Alto, CA: Science and Behavior Books. Grinder, J., & Bandler, R. (1976). *The structure of magic* (Vol. II). Palo Alto, CA: Science and Behavior Books.
6. Kahneman, D. (2017). *Thinking, fast and slow.* Farrar, Straus and Giroux.
7. Bargh, J. (2017). *Before you know it: The unconscious reasons we do what we do.* Simon and Schuster.

8. Newcombe, N. S., Drummey, A. B., Fox, N. A., Lie, E., & Ottinger-Alberts, W. (2000). Remembering early childhood: How much, how, and why (or why not). *Current directions in psychological science, 9*(2), 55–58.
9. Karen, R. (1998). *Becoming attached: First relationships and how they shape our capacity to love.* Oxford University Press, USA.
10. Bowlby, J. *Attachment,* 1969; *Separation: Anxiety and Anger,* 1972; *Loss: Sadness and Depression,* 1980. Random House.
11. Spitz, R. A. (1946). Hospitalism: A follow-up report on investigation described in Volume I, 1945. *The psychoanalytic study of the child, 2*(1), 113–117.
12. Karen, R. (1998). *Becoming attached: First relationships and how they shape our capacity to love.* Oxford University Press, USA.
13. http://www.aaimhiwa.org/store/p16/Young_Children_in_Brief_Separation_%22John%22_DVD.html.
14. Kaler, S. R., & Freeman, B. J. (1994). Analysis of environmental deprivation: Cognitive and social development in Romanian orphans. *Journal of Child Psychology and Psychiatry, 35*(4), 769–781.
15. Porges, S. W. (2011). *The polyvagal theory: Neurophysiological foundations of emotions, attachment, communication, and self-regulation (Norton Series on Interpersonal Neurobiology).* WW Norton & Company.
16. Dawkins, R. (2016). *The selfish gene.* Oxford university press.
17. Vetere, A., & Dallos, R. (2008). Systemic therapy and attachment narratives. *Journal of Family Therapy, 30*(4), 374–385.
18. Dallos, R., & Vetere, A. (2021). *Systemic therapy and attachment narratives: Applications in a range of clinical settings.* Routledge.
19. Dallos, R. (2006). Attachment Narrative Therapy: Integrating Narrative, Systemic and Attachment Therapies. United Kingdom: McGraw-Hill Education; Dallos, R., Vetere, A. (2021). Systemic Therapy and Attachment Narratives: Applications in a Range of Clinical Settings. United Kingdom: Taylor & Francis.
20. Dallos, R., & Vetere, A. (2021). *Systemic therapy and attachment narratives: Applications in a range of clinical settings.* Routledge.
21. Carnes, P. (2001). *Out of the shadows: Understanding sexual addiction.* Hazelden Publishing.
22. Carnes, P. J., Delmonico, D. L., & Griffin, E. (2009). *In the shadows of the net: Breaking free of compulsive online sexual behavior.* Simon and Schuster. Carnes, P. J. (2018, August). *Betrayal Bond, Revised: Breaking Free of Exploitive Relationships.* Hci. Carnes, P. (2013). *Don't call it love: Recovery from sexual addiction.* Bantam. And others.

CHAPTER 2

Maslow's Modified Hierarchy

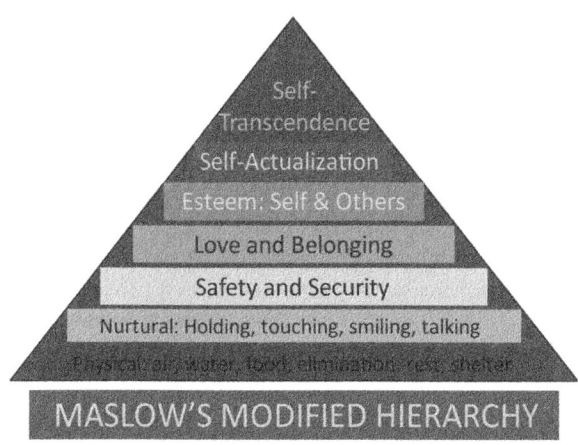

Abraham Maslow identified our needs in his eponymous hierarchy.[1] Bowlby identified the Attachment Behavioural System (ABS) by which those needs are met. In ACT, attachment theory and Maslow's Modified Hierarchy (MMH) go hand in hand. MMH gives us a specific progression of levels that are not age-specific, contrary to other developmental models.[2]

C. Shults, *Attachment Centred Therapy*, Palgrave Texts in Counselling and Psychotherapy, https://doi.org/10.1007/978-3-031-60851-3_2

Maslow's view of humanity was based on growth and possibility, or the idea of wellness, as reflected in the titles of his books such as *The Farther Reaches of Human Nature*.[3] He thought that it would be better to study what helped people to thrive and fulfil their potential rather than what made them pathological. His vision was an alternative to either system in vogue at the time.[4] Those two were the psychoanalytic tradition of Freud and others, and the 'black box' approach of the behaviourists.

Maslow's vision was different. His view of human beings was that we are driven by our needs. In that sense, he was a harbinger of attachment theory. Maslow viewed human development as our effort to be our best selves. As I interpret Maslow, anything less than that is attributable to a failure to meet needs at lower levels so that the higher levels are continually undercut.

From an attachment perspective, we have already looked at the need for physical survival. We are dependent on our caregivers for the things we need to stay alive: the physiological needs. As Spitz and others research established, we also need nurturing or the second level of attachment needs. This failure of nurturing can lead to death, but even if it doesn't, it does impair in other ways, including our ability to form satisfying relationships with ourselves and with others. Likewise, parental inattention can lead to offspring being killed and eaten or dying from other threatening causes: drowning, avalanches, landslides, etc.

Maslow wrote of our needs in general.[5] Specifically, he said there were 'at least' five basic needs: physiological, safety, love, esteem, and self-actualization. Maslow wanted to have a more spiritual title for self-actualization, but he was afraid that such a term would turn off the psychological establishment of the time since it had adopted a reductionistic belief system, so he borrowed the term from Kurt Goldstein[6] that was already acceptable.

He later came to regret the choice. Some people seize on the 'self' in self-actualization and misunderstand it as 'selfish.' This is wildly incorrect. Self-actualization is about making your best contribution to the good of humankind. Self-actualization is inherently altruistic and is based on helping others, not selfishly pursuing one's own interests to the detriment of others. This is readily understood when we consider the extent to which each level affects others favourably: the higher we go, the more people we reach.

The misunderstanding is perhaps in part because self-actualized people go their own way. They aren't too concerned about whom they may offend or what rubrics they might violate. While they are not necessarily contrarians, they are not afraid to go against the prevailing belief systems.

I have come to Maslow's rescue in this regard by giving 'Self-Actualization' an alternative name: spiritual awakening. Maslow's idea here is the same as that expressed by many spiritual teachers that the higher you go, the more you serve.[7]

I have further modified Maslow's Hierarchy by making two additions. I did not make these additions arbitrarily, but rather, in response to client needs and feelings, appropriately enough for a surrogate attachment relationship.

In my modified form the hierarchy is: physical, nurtural, safety and security, love and belonging, esteem of self and others, self-actualization/ spiritual wakening, and self-transcendence. I believe that Maslow would agree with my modifications.

PHYSICAL

Briefly, at the physical level of need, we are only concerned about our own individual survival. As long as we have air to breath, water to drink, food to eat, elimination of waste, rest for recuperation, and shelter, we will survive absent some cause of death. It is only concerned with individual survival. We are, of course, better able to meet these needs when we cooperate with others. Even bacteria and slime mould have been observed doing that. Shelter is optional in that some environments are benign and shelter is not necessary for survival. But even then, to have shelter, a place that we call home, is comforting. It can be a physical manifestation of an emotional need.

In terms of attachment, this is where it is essential for the parents to teach the child good self-care. This is also where emotional disorders, such as eating, can find a place in the mind's desire to get those feelings and reassurances: this feels good and everything is going to be all right.[8] Food feels good because the things that promote our wellbeing *do* feel good. In that regard, Freud was right. We do have a drive to survive, to reproduce, to thrive.

NURTURAL

In working with clients using an A5 Compulsive Promiscuity Sexual strategy and also the C6 Punitive Strategy, I realized the need to separate the nurturing needs from the physical needs. There are several reasons for this separation. First, as a practical matter, to approach sexuality with those who are using it compulsively as if it were a need similar to air, water, food, and so on, would only reinforce their core belief of sex being essential for survival. Second, you don't *necessarily* die if your nurturing needs are not met. But as Spitz and others have made clear, it *can* result in death. That is why it is such a powerful drive and why it trumps the need for safety and security.

This is the level of reproduction and families. It is the essence of the attachment bond. When we don't have adequate nurturing, we cannot thrive and sometimes we don't survive.

In attachment terms, this is where we learn how to have attachment relationships. In infancy and early childhood, the brain is being rapidly wired and the mind rapidly programmed to adapt to the environment. In fact, there is abundant evidence that this process begins in the womb.[9] When we have a close, nurturing relationship with our attachment figures, then we develop the neurology and beliefs to accommodate that and later to reproduce it when we enter our own mating and reproduction phase. We also develop a robust sense of self-worth so that when life gives us setbacks, we don't take it personally. We are resilient, and we are able to be vulnerable and to ask others for help.

When we don't have those interactions that create secure attachment, then we are left feeling worth less than others. The different strategies respond to this shame in different ways. Those using the 'A' strategy by being preoccupied with the needs and feelings of others and dismissive of their own, and those using the 'C' strategy by being preoccupied with their own needs and feelings and dismissive of the needs and feelings of others. Those using the 'B' strategy are going to work cooperatively and communicate effectively out of the realization that they will be able to get their own needs met best by helping others to get their needs met. That is the basis of progress upwards through the hierarchy!

> *We meet our own needs best*
> *When we help others meet their needs best*

I will sometimes refer to A's, B's, and C's. That is for convenience. Please understand that what I mean is that they are using that strategy. Although this may be what generally happens, the clients I see are often using an A/C strategy that combines behaviours of both A and C. They may switch strategies depending on who they are relating to or in different circumstances.

SAFETY AND SECURITY

Next, we have the need to protect ourselves and our offspring: the ones in whom we have invested so much time and energy nurturing. We discover that we can do this better if we have allies. Other families combine with ours for our mutual defence against predators, hostile humans, natural disasters, and so on. We got so good at protecting ourselves from predators that we have got rid of most of them. We organized ourselves into bands, tribes, states, nations, alliances. This organization, increasing as we encounter more threat, in turn creating more threat, in an escalating manner, has brought us where we are today. We have got so good at protecting ourselves from enemies that we are now in the position of being able to kill off virtually everyone on any given day. 'We have met the enemy, and [they are] us.'[10] We humans are now the biggest threat to life that we face.

We also live in a dangerous world. Protection from danger is paramount. No matter how good a job of parenting you have done, if your offspring dies you have failed to reproduce successfully. If you don't have one who does survive to reproduce, then your particular genetic legacy is at an end. Of course, most parents have multiple offspring, but no one wants to experience the death of a child.

We also have the threats from caregivers themselves. As cases such as Baby P,[11] Victoria Climbie,[12] Susan Smith,[13] and Andrea Yates[14] illustrate, sometimes the greatest threat we face *is* our parent. When we don't feel safe with our caregivers, then it makes it difficult to be vulnerable, not only with them but with others to whom we are connected as attachment figures. Hence:

> *We need to feel safe*
> *With the people we need*
> *To feel safe.*

Lest we fall into the smug assumption that these dangerous parents were simply monstrous aberrations, we need to remember that these parents were once children as well and that they, too, were subjected to abuse and a failure of nurturing. And, forgive me for saying it, these children would have been much more susceptible to becoming abusive parents themselves. Trauma, abuse, and neglect can be handed down, like family heirlooms, from one generation to the next.

Not only that, entire cultures can be based on fear and anger due to a lack of safety and security needs being met. (In this regard, see Turchin[15] and his concept of asabiyya.[16]).

When we do get our needs for safety and security met, then we can move to the next level.

LOVE AND BELONGING

Fortunately, we have also noticed that one way to reduce threat is to get what we want by trade and negotiation. From the previous level of mutual defence and assistance, affectional bonds are created. We realize that if we can arrange to trade with others who have what we want and who want what we have, then that is a much better way to make a living than waging war against one another. Now we have a genuine sense of community. Originally, this was defined geographically. Today communities are much more inclusive and dispersed so that we can have worldwide communities. And, indeed, many of the challenges we face are worldwide.

In attachment terms, at this level we are motivated to form bonds with others based on positive feelings. Instead of escaping death at the first level, escaping shame at the second level, and escaping fear at the third level, we are seeking pleasure in association with others. We transition from physical survival needs to more intangible needs. It is where we seek gain rather than avoid loss.

This means being willing to take risks with your loved one. It also eliminates the confusion of identifying love and loving actions strictly with a pleasurable reward. While it will ultimately lead to pleasure, in the near term it may mean being able to tolerate difficult feelings without being reactive. Rather, to seek to deal with those difficult feelings by understanding them and seeking to work together to meet the unmet needs giving rise to the feelings.

The definition of love as we use it here is from Scott Peck, *The Road Less Travelled*:

> *Love is being willing*
> *To extend yourself*
> *For the spiritual growth*
> *Of yourself and others.*[17]

ESTEEM OF SELF AND OTHERS

Communities cooperating with one another then lead us to our esteem needs. We admire an article of clothing that far exceeds anything we have seen before. We want to know who made it. We learn that it was made by someone far away and only came to us via trade routes (or we found it on Amazon). Meantime, someone else is admiring the atlatl that we made with a new innovation (or the new algorithm we created). Thus, we may earn the respect and admiration of someone far away whom we may never meet. Or we may be a great war leader whose reputation is known far and wide or a great peacemaker who is held in great esteem. Esteem is based on what we contribute to others. It is based on the respect and admiration that we earn with our deeds, our skills, our willingness to serve others.

In attachment terms, when we are secure, we can accept our own accomplishments with graciousness and our failures with equanimity. Our self-worth is secure because it is based on robust accomplishment (a secure relationship) at the nurturing level. We can celebrate the successes of others without feeling threat or jealousy. We can genuinely enjoy their accomplishments and even contribute to them.

When we are insecure, even great achievements can leave us wanting and empty: the 'imposter syndrome.' We don't believe we are worthy of the accolades. We expect we will be exposed as frauds at any moment. We vainly seek more and more external accomplishments to compensate for our low opinion of ourselves. This idea is at the basis of the Groucho effect: I refuse to belong to any club that would have someone like me as a member!

SELF-ACTUALIZATION/SPIRITUAL AWAKENING

Next, we come to self-actualization aka spiritual awakening. This is the philosophical stance that we serve ourselves best when we serve others. This philosophy is found in all major philosophical systems. Maslow continues this tradition in this humanistic version of philosophy.

In attachment terms, this means being willing and able to reach out to others, to contribute what we have to offer for the benefit of humanity. When I use the term 'spirit,' I refer to the spirit of life that exists within us all.

SELF-TRANSCENDENCE

Finally is self-transcendence about which Maslow wrote extensively. Transpersonal Psychology is a manifestation of his ideas about self-transcendence, as is this modified hierarchy. Maslow spoke of 'peak experiences,' and associated those with self-actualization/spiritual awakening. However, I think that it belongs more properly in the self-transcendence level. The two terms suggest that their essence is about going beyond the ordinary, everyday level of experience, even if that level, that is self-actualization/spiritual awakening, is itself extraordinary.

These needs are homogenous. Separating them into distinct categories, while useful, can also be misleading if we think of them as rungs on a ladder that we reach one at a time. Rather, we must think of them as phases, or vibrations, much as the notes of a musical composition, that come in and out as the tapestry is woven.

NOTES

1. Maslow, A. (1974). *A theory of human motivation*. Lulu.com.
2. Erikson, E. (1959). Theory of identity development. *E. Erikson, Identity and the life cycle. Nueva York: International Universities Press. Obtenido de http://childdevpsychology. Yolasite. com/resources/theory% 20of% 20ident ity% 20erikson. pdf*. Huitt, W., & Hummel, J. (2003). Piaget's theory of cognitive development. *Educational psychology interactive, 3*(2).
3. Maslow, A. H. (1971). *The farther reaches of human nature* (Vol. 19,711). New York: Viking Press.
4. Goble, F. G. (1970). *The third force: The psychology of Abraham Maslow*. Grossman.
5. Maslow, A. H. (1954). *Motivation and Personality by AH Maslow*. Prabhat Prakashan.
6. Maslow, A. (1974). *A theory of human motivation*. Lulu.com.
7. Mathew, 23–11, Christian Bible.
8. Milkman, H. B., & Sunderwirth, S. G. (1998). *Craving for ecstasy: How our passions become addictions and what we can do about them*. Sage.
9. Cerritelli, F., Frasch, M. G., Antonelli, M. C., Viglione, C., Vecchi, S., Chiera, M., & Manzotti, A. (2021). A review on the vagus nerve and autonomic nervous system during fetal development: searching for critical windows. *Frontiers in Neuroscience, 15*, 721,605. Emory, E. K. (2010). A womb with a view: Ultrasound for evaluation of fetal neurobehavioral development. *Infant and Child Development: An International Journal of Research and Practice, 19*(1), 119–124.

10. https://www.dictionary.com/browse/we-have-met-the-enemy%2D%
    2Dand-they-are-us.
11. https://www.theguardian.com/society/2009/aug/16/baby-p-family.
12. https://www.gov.uk/government/publications/the-victoria-climbie-
    inquiry-report-of-an-inquiry-by-lord-laming.
13. https://en.wikipedia.org/wiki/Susan_Smith.
14. https://allthatsinteresting.com/andrea-yates.
15. Turchin, P. (2005). *War and peace and war: The life cycles of imperial nations.* New York: Pi.
16. Sümer, B. (2012). Ibn Khaldun's asabiyya for social cohesion. *Elektronik Sosyal Bilimler Dergisi, 11*(41), 253–267.
17. Peck, M. S. (2002). *The road less traveled: A new psychology of love, traditional values, and spiritual growth.* Simon and Schuster.

CHAPTER 3

The Dynamic Maturational Model of Attachment

When offered the chance to move to England to help establish a treatment centre, I gladly accepted. I was looking to get out of Alabama for reasons that current events make glaringly obvious. Helping to start a treatment centre would pay for my move across the Atlantic, give me a chance to incorporate attachment theory into treating addictively disordered behaviours, and establish a reputation and a start on clientele for my private practice when my 2-year contract ended. I ran the family programme and the trauma programme. Both were week-long programmes and they gave me the opportunity to begin to apply this new knowledge of attachment. When I began my private practice, I thought of it as Attachment Centred Therapy. I would use the skills and experience that I had already gained combined with attachment theory, the 'missing link,' as I had already discovered. I thought that would be an ideal arrangement.

Central was attachment, attended by a variety of other therapies that would address the psychodynamic, cognitive/behavioural, and affective aspects of behaviour. It would be a full spectrum approach to helping clients meet their needs and deal with their feelings effectively, repairing the damage done by their insecure relationships in the past.

I experimented. I found the Experiences in Close Relationships[1] questionnaire online and began to use it. It was quick and easy to administer and score, and I created an Excel spreadsheet to display the results. I

© The Author(s), under exclusive license to Springer Nature Switzerland AG 2024
C. Shults, *Attachment Centred Therapy*, Palgrave Texts in Counselling and Psychotherapy,
https://doi.org/10.1007/978-3-031-60851-3_3

created a third scale, 'confusion v. certainty,' to go with the two original scales, and created a three dimensional model of it. It was easy for clients to see and understand. Too easy, it turns out.

It was easy for clients to fool. The questions are quite obvious, and so anyone who is motivated to give misleading information can do so quite easily. Also, if people are fooling themselves, when someone really believes what they are saying, no matter how divergent from reality it is, there is no way to know. It is also very dependent on current circumstances. For example, people who have been in a stable relationship for some time are going to give a certain impression no matter how miserable they may be in the relationship. In other words, the advantages were also disadvantages. It also yielded little insight into the intrapsychic dynamics of the person. And last but not least, the most effective deception is sincere. I don't presume that people come to pay me money in order to fool me—although some do! No, they are paying to fool themselves and maintain their illusions. Also, despite the description, the instrument only measures romantic relationships, not the original parental relationships. And people, especially those seeking therapy, often use multiple strategies depending on circumstances.

Next, I tried the BABI (Brief Attachment Based Inventory) from Jeremy Holmes book, *The Search for the Secure Base*.[2] I copied the inventory into a Word format and, as intended, gave it to the clients to complete. That was a dud. The AAI is not valid if given to the client to provide written answers. Clients will second-guess and edit their answers. The dysfluency that accompanies thinking spontaneously will be missing. Discrepancies will be noted and corrected. In short, all the important information on which coding is based will be missing.

Although I was successfully using the concept of attachment and the A, B, and C categories, I knew I needed to learn more about it. As I continued to read the available literature, I found something very confusing to me. That was the 'disorganized' category. Studies were being reported using the 'three-factor model,' A, B, and C, and the 'four-factor model' A, B, C, and D. (They use different nomenclature for adult relationships that, to add to the confusion, do not proceed in sequence: Ds—dismissing; F—free, autonomous; and E—enmeshed.)

Then I learned about 'the transmission gap.' It is a fiction they needed to create because reality does not match their assumptions. Rather than discard the erroneous assumptions, they have been attempting to find this elusive missing factor in 'transmitting' the strategy to the child. Unable to find this will-o-the-wisp, they have created another assumption. This 'transmission gap' was based on a series of fundamental errors. The first and most egregious error was the *assumption* that the mother's attachment strategy would be passed along to her child. Then, in the absence of any adverse childhood experiences, it would remain the same until adulthood. That child would then have children to whom they would 'transmit' the same attachment strategy.

This did not make sense to me. It was painfully obvious based on my own childhood and my siblings and their families that this theory did not conform to reality. Nor was it even close, even with the limited knowledge that I had, to being able to describe the reality of my clients' experiences. That is when I decided to invest the time and money to get formal training in using the AAI. Luckily for me and my clients, that is when I found Pat Crittenden and the Dynamic Maturational Model.

The three basic patterns: A, B, and C, were formulated by Bowlby with his student and later, colleague, Mary Salter Ainsworth, based on observations in the Strange Situation Procedure (SSP).[3] These were further subdivided into A1–2, B1–4 (later B1–5), and C1–2. Two of Ainsworth's students and then colleagues developed the model further into two rather different models. First was the ABC+D, or Berkeley Model, of Mary Main, et al. and the second was the Dynamic Maturational Model of Patricia Crittenden, et al., or DMM. It is this later model, the DMM, that we will be using in this book. The reason that I am using the DMM is because it is far and away the best, in my opinion.

Both these models retained the original Ainsworth patterns. The D in the ABC+D model was added by Mary Main. This stands for 'Disorganized.' This is a catchall category for anything that does not fit in the original Ainsworth categories, except for some categories added at the C-3 and A-3 levels. This was based on the assumption that safety organizes and danger disorganizes. It has led to disastrous consequences.[4] (The footnoted article was written by the very researchers who spread the D category initially and are still trying to rehabilitate it. The confusion this has created has led to dead ends in research and unfortunately informs many professionals' low opinions of attachment theory's efficacy.[5,6] In the first reference, the title as given in Google Scholar is misleading. In the *BPS*

Journal the title is, 'Overrated: The Predictive Power of Attachment.' In the latter reference, *The Myth of Attachment Theory,* the author actually makes some very good points critical of the ABC+D model of attachment. Specifically, regarding the role of alternative sources of attachment security and cultural variations on how children are raised. It would have been useful if she had contrasted the ABC+D model with the DMM, but neither referenced author apparently knows that the DMM exists.)

Crittenden took the contrary view. She maintains that danger organizes. She is right. Imagine that you are a member of village that comes under attack unexpectedly. Of course, you will be disorganized, running around like the proverbial headless chicken. But you manage to survive the attack. Now what are you going to do? Are you going to helplessly await the next attack? No. You are going to eventually organize yourself to deal with the threat. You are going to become much more organized. But unfortunately, not always in a way that is helpful for you. That is, it helps to meet the present threat, but when circumstances change the strategy may be counterproductive. One need only look at the present situation in Ukraine and ask if the Ukrainians have become more or less organized. One need only look at the history of Russia to understand their dysfunctional organization around perceived threat.

As Rudi Dallos observes, organized is not the same as functional. As I understand the term 'dysfunctional,' it refers to not operating normally or optimally. In the addiction treatment world, we would routinely refer to dysfunctional relationships and families. This was informed by a particular world view of what 'functional' would be. As treatment centres are not centres of mental and emotional health, we generally defined functional as 'not dysfunctional.' These families became highly organized in order to deal with the dysfunctional dilemmas presented by addictively disordered behaviour.

In viewing these children in the SSP whose behaviour could not be categorized as one of the already existing categories, Mary Main saw them as anomalies, or 'disorganized,' hence the label. Crittenden saw them as discrepant from the previously established categories and theorized that there was valuable, essential information to be had from understanding these discrepancies. Out of Crittenden's approach, the DMM was born. It currently looks like this:

The Dynamic Maturational Model of Attachment:[7]

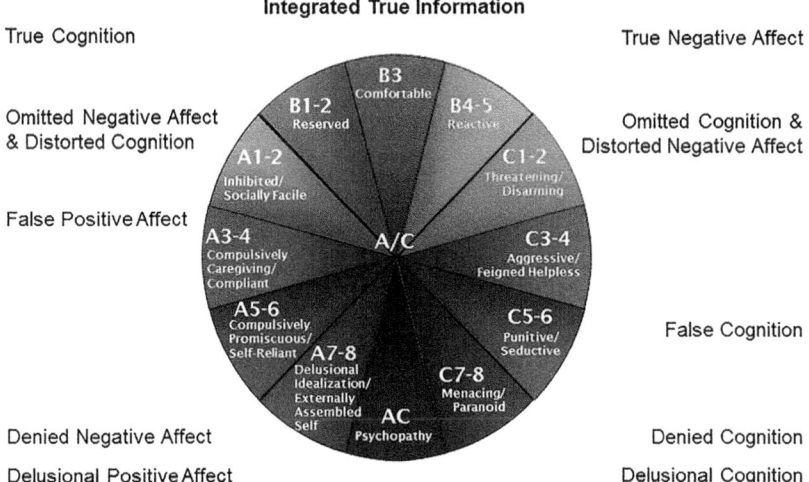

As you can see from this model, our original A, B, and C designations have been extended and refined. It is in the nature of evolutionary models that they extend themselves and refine themselves.[8]

I recommend that you follow the link to Crittenden's website,[9] where, under 'DMM Model,' you will find an interactive version of this chart. You can read the descriptions of the various categories. They are extremely useful. I often go to this website with my clients and look at the various categories. We talk about which categories they might be using. We discuss what this would mean in terms of the client's issues that brought them into therapy. And we can do this at any time that it might be useful to calibrate ourselves to the model. I suggest that you familiarize yourself with the categories because we will be referring to them a good deal going through the stories and interventions later on. You may even want to bookmark the page for easy reference.

I have created a comparison chart for the two models in Appendix A. As you can see, the ABC+D model has only about half of the categories that the DMM has. And they stop at or before the halfway point. Everything in the bottom part of the DMM is dumped into the D category in the ABC+D. This includes virtually all the classifications that are of clinical interest. It is, in cartographic terms, the equivalent of 'Here Be Dragons!' It includes virtually everyone who will come to us for help. It includes A3–8 (A+), C3–8 (C+) and AC, or psychopathy. AC should not to be confused with A/C which is the designation used for mixed strategies. Mixed strategies may consist of alternating, blended, conflicting, and layered.

THE ADULT ATTACHMENT INTERVIEW

The Adult Attachment Interview is the beating heart of ACT. Specifically, the DMM-AAI: it has been significantly modified and its interpretation extended into new territory by Crittenden. The AAI has been found to have high validity and reliability in test/retest.[10] This is remarkable considering that it is a semi-structured interview that elicits information from the interviewee about their childhood. It asks about one's earliest memories, about relationships with attachment figures, how certain fairly universal topics were handled, how threatening situations were handled, how things have changed, and how they are now. It can stir up things from the past dramatically, and so people who take the interview need to be supported emotionally.

The AAI provides a way of understanding the subtle and sometimes not so subtle ways that clients' information processing was developed and where it is distorted. It allows us to understand how clients have adapted themselves to their world. Some clients describe experiencing the interview process as transformative in itself, because of the way it asks the speaker to think about their attachment relationships.

The DMM-AAI has been modified from the original by Crittenden to make certain improvements in the flow of information. In addition, I have made certain changes that suit my own purposes. The original asks about the childhood relationship with parents. This was changed substantially by Crittenden. First, she asks about the parents separately instead of as a unit. Alfred Adler in his theory of parenting advised that the parents be united in their interactions with children. He maintained that the worst kind of parenting was to have one who was authoritarian and the other permissive. Crittenden's change recognizes this and probes the relationship with each parent separately. She has also changed the word 'adjectives' to 'words or phrases' to reflect that not everyone understands the word 'adjectives,' but everyone does understand 'words or phrases.' I have further altered my version by alternating the questions between mom and dad. That is, I ask the first question about mom and then about dad. Then I do the same for the second question and then the third. What I observed is that often the interviewee, having heard all three questions for mom immediately before, then gets the questions conflated in their mind, so that for dad they will often, when asked the first question, respond to the second question instead because they have just recently heard it and so they anticipate it coming. I think my method works nicely and I have never had a problem with it, and it eliminates the problem of the interviewee getting confused about which question they are answering.

In working with the AAI, there are several aspects with which one needs to be familiar. First is the AAI protocol. Too much deviation from this protocol will interfere with reliable coding. Second are the follow-up questions—whether and how much is a judgement call. Third is transcribing of the interview. This needs to be done by someone following the correct protocol that means as many of the nuances of expression are captured as possible. Pauses, stutters, restarts, and so on, need to be reproduced in the transcript as accurately as possible, as well as any somatic expressions such as yawning, coughing, etc. In addition, I like to have the actual recording of the interview so that, in case of doubt, I can listen to it.

ADMINISTER THE ADULT ATTACHMENT INTERVIEW

The interview setting needs to be where interruptions are unlikely. I set aside 3 hours for the interview, but I only charge for the amount of time actually used. The original use of the AAI was for research purposes and was intended to be done in 1–1.5 hours. For ACT, I am interested in much more than merely arriving at a classification. For that reason, I usually let the client talk for as long as they wish to answer any given question. Giving the interview is a way to get to know my client. Because the information is what we will be working on, then I want to get it as early as possible. Because the interview is structured, it keeps the information contextual rather than unstructured rambling about the past.

I record the interview and make a backup recording in case something happens to the primary. Next is transcription. Specialized knowledge is required. Instead of 'cleaning up' the recording, the aim is to capture as many of the nuances of non-verbal expression as possible. These are dysfluencies.

Dysfluency is like a disturbance of the flow of water. By looking at the surface of the water in a river, we can deduce what is underneath. If we see a smoothly flowing surface, we can reasonably infer that there is nothing particularly noteworthy underneath. The more agitated the water, the more obstruction underneath. In the same way, we can analyse the discourse in order to get an 'x-ray vision' idea of what is going on in the client's mind.

CODING THE TRANSCRIPT

When you get the transcript back, the first thing you are going to need to do is to read through it. At this point, if you have been through the DMM-AAI training, you will know how to code and classify. If you haven't yet had it, you can find available trainings on Dr. Crittenden's website.[11] Your best reference source for this information is *Assessing Adult Attachment: A Dynamic-Maturational Approach to Discourse Analysis,* by Crittenden and Landini.[12]

Next comes the coding of the transcript. This consists of identifying 'discourse markers' that are associated with the various strategies. When you decide to train with Dr. Crittenden or one of her trainers, you will receive a deep immersion into these discourse markers and the codes associated with each. The final step is to arrive at a classification based on the patterns created by the discourse markers. Just as individual pixels make up an electronic photograph, so do the discourse markers create a 'picture' or model of the world that the client is using.

Once you understand discourse markers and can identify them, you will be able to incorporate them more and more into your therapy sessions. As you acquaint your clients with their particular discourse markers, they will be able to begin to identify them in real time and can change their discourse, hence their information processing, in real time.

What follows are the various concepts that go into coding. This is not an attempt to teach you about them, but rather to let you know the dazzling array of tools that will be at your disposal once you learn how to code. They are: Grice's Maxims, Childhood History, Dispositional Representations (DRs), and Discourse Markers. We will look at each of these in turn.

Grice's Maxims

The most basic concept is Grice's Maxims.[13] They are the first and most important and they are easy to understand and apply. They are essential to what Grice called 'the cooperative principle.' We (almost all of us[14]) use these maxims automatically in order to communicate and cooperate.

Relevance
This is the most immediate of the maxims, I think, because if information is not relevant to us, then we are going to ignore it or perhaps be annoyed or puzzled. If I ask you what you want to achieve in life and you start talking about the hula hoop craze, then I am going to wonder what the relevance is. In the same way, if I ask a client to tell me about their childhood growing up and they start telling me about guidance systems for nuclear submarines and how a family vacation got cancelled, then I am going to be puzzled, because it doesn't seem relevant to the question. If I query what the relevance is, the speaker may reply that the reason they have problems was their father spent all his time at the shipyard and neglected them. I can then understand the tangential relevance. Most important, I have some very strong clues as to the speaker's attachment strategy: C+.

The first clue is that the information is not clearly relevant to the query. We can get the relevance *to the speaker*, but the speaker has not mentalized in order to anticipate that their answer will not be apparently relevant nor will it answer the question.

The second clue is that when the speaker does make the connection for us, they reduce it to the single factor that is causing their problems today, so that is probably going to be reductionist blaming thought. All the variables in creating who they are today are attributed to their father's behaviour towards work.

Third is the use of absolutes: dad spent *all* his time at the shipyard and that is the *only* reason for *all* the client's problems today.

So the relevance of relevance at this point is that it is one of the most important and easily understood of the discourse markers. It is also something that we therapists need to keep in mind as we work with our clients. Is what I am saying relevant to their problem? Is what they are saying relevant to my enquiry?

Manner
Manner is the *way* in which the information is presented. Is the manner conducive to understanding? Clients using an A strategy will generally give factual information, quite concise. For example, 'Born in Glasgow, moved to London when I was 4.' Or they might give a rather long and detailed description of the houses in which they lived in each location. But no

emotion. A client using a C strategy might say: 'Well, my parents wanted to be close to their parents so that they could help with raising us kids, so we all grew up together in a neighbourhood that had been there for a long time. And my mother, well, her grandmother was ill when I was born so she had to help take care of her, but then my father had to go to London for a new job. So when we moved there I had to make new friends all over again and I didn't like it because my old friends—well, I mean, they weren't *old,* if you see what I mean. I mean, they were the same age as me, of course, which is why we were friends. (laughs) Well, not friends really, but I didn't mind too much because there was lots more to do in London. But then when I went to University.'

That is an example of the micro meaning of manner. The macro meaning is, overall, how comprehensible is the client's disposition of their reality? Can we understand it and make sense of it? Is it coherent? Fluid? Or do they obfuscate? Contradict? Become frustrated with all these questions? Are they cooperative? Combative? Obsequious? These are factors in how they relate to the interviewer, which is one of the most important discourse markers.

Quantity

Next is quantity. This refers to both the length and depth of information conveyed, and I suppose we might add width as well. It is sometimes called the Goldilocks principle. We don't want too much or too little, too hot or too cold, too hard or too soft, but rather, just right. It is one of the things that aspiring writers must contend with!

I am reminded of the joke about the farmer and his wife. His wife was ill and couldn't go to church that Sunday, so the farmer went alone. When he got home, his wife asked him, 'What was the sermon about today?' The farmer replied, 'Sin.' The wife was understandably annoyed at such a brief answer. 'Well,' she demanded, 'what did the preacher say about it?' The farmer replied, 'He were agin' it.'

This is an example of too little information, a clue to the farmer's A+ strategy. A6 could be a very adaptive strategy for a farmer!

If the situation was reversed, however, the wife, if we hypothesize the A and C dichotomy that many couples exhibit, might have come home, late, and without waiting to be asked proceed to tell not only all about the sermon but about Sister Lulabelle's best heifer getting sick and dying, Sister Mildred's cousin's son getting arrested on a drunk driving charge, and oh by the way, did he know that Simon Henderson had died and that they already had the funeral but his youngest son couldn't be there because he was stationed in Korea and there wasn't time for him to fly home before the funeral.

Quality

Next is quality. This goes to the truth of what is being said. Is there evidence to support the point being made? Is it consistent with what we know to be true? That is why you will find, I hope, throughout this book, references that support the points being made.

Likewise, when working with clients, I give them references to provide evidence for what I am saying. This could be in the form of books, articles, or videos online. When I am deciding whether or not to use a particular therapy, I want to know whether or not there is any particular body of research, practice, or observation to support it.

Summary

These maxims are both an indicator of attachment strategies and also a means of correcting the errors of information. These maxims are always at play in our interactions with our clients. Like defence mechanisms, we can bring them into conscious awareness and give ourselves choice over whether we use them or not.

According to Crittenden and Landini,[15] there are three sources of information that are used in the coding and classifying of the interview. They are childhood history of life events, memory systems or 'dispositional representations,' and discourse markers.[16] Lacking better terminology, I will refer to all these collectively as 'discourse markers.' The first is the 'childhood history of life events.'

Childhood History

This is the most obvious aspect. This is what gets our attention most easily and conveniently. When we give the interview, the questions are directed towards describing the important and also the day-to-day events in the life of the child that the adult once was. As pointed out earlier, a life story that seems, on the surface, quite idealistic (typically the A strategy) often masks a life that was disturbingly non-nurturing. Idealizing clients will often distort information by making it seem better than it actually was. On the other hand, tales of horror are sometimes exaggerations that reflect a tendency to make things seem worse than they really were, typically the C strategy. And sometimes, clients will give quite horrific stories that have veracity, but because of how those events have been dealt with between then and now, the client is resolved regarding them, and so has the potential to be balanced, though you are unlikely to see them in therapy: typically the B strategy.

The obvious recounting of events may not be what actually happened when we examine it. Yet how the client relates the event in conjunction with what actually happened gives us information about their information processing. How do we know the obvious information isn't entirely accurate?

Well, we don't yet. This is where the analysis and the discourse markers come into play. We look for discrepancies in the dialogue. (There will be some good ones presented early on. See if you can spot them. Clues: ducking books and severed digits.) The authors list the following as 'constructs' of childhood history:

1. Comfort—this refers to whether or not the parent provided comfort for negative feelings. So, for example, if the child says, 'Mommy, I'm scared,' and Mommy replies, 'Oh, don't be silly. There's nothing to be scared of,' that's not comforting, is it? It's dismissing.

2. Protection—To continue with the previous example, Mommy may not be comforting, but she may be protective. Hence, her message of 'There's nothing to be scared of,' might quite literally be true, in her mind, because 'I'm here to protect you.' Comfort and protection are two different things, not mutually exclusive but far from synonymous.

3. Danger—Here I shall refer to my saying, 'We need to feel safe with the people we need to feel safe.' The most obvious aspect of danger is that the world is a dangerous place, and our parents are the source of protection from that danger, literally. But there also needs to be the *perception* of safety from danger. It's bad enough when children don't feel safe because they don't perceive that they are protected from danger by their parents. But what's worse is when the parents *are the biggest threat that the child faces!* This is the classic double bind: you're not safe with them, you're not safe without them.

4. Rejection—My Mom gave me the best example of this one. I remember as a child attempting to express my anger with her. Her

response, 'If you're going to be angry you can't be my boy.' The effect on me was dramatic. I instantly had an intense feeling of dread that dictated to me that I conform to her wishes. On another occasion, I was beaten so badly by my father, at her instigation, that I *wanted* to be abandoned. I remember thinking that if they would just stop the car and let me out, I would go down into the cabbage patch and live under the cabbage leaves with the rabbits, and the rabbits would take care of me. It may have been the thought of a constant diet of cabbage leaves that dissuaded me!

5. Involvement—This has to do with what in other circles is known as 'boundaries' and 'boundary violations.' There are various 'involvements' that can occur. These are:

a. Parent joins sibling subsystem—this is where one of the parents becomes more like a child themselves, leaving the other parent to do the parenting, or where the parent and child become 'best mates,' the parent eschewing parental responsibility.

b. 'Affect contagion' where the parent 'empathizes' with the child to such an extent that they can no longer be effective parents. This leaves the child without adult guidance as to how to label the emotion, and worse, how to deal with it effectively. Both child and adult are swept along on the winds of emotion.

c. Involving: all these examples, or types, are characterized by lack of appropriate boundaries:

 i. Competitive—in this case, the parent competes with the child inappropriately. Crittenden and Landini limit their examples to receiving 'attention, caregiving and comfort.' I shall add that competition can also extend to performance competition where the parent enhances their own fragile ego by beating the child in 'friendly' competition at games and other play. Or more lately, reading of the mother of the groom who wears what looks suspiciously like a wedding dress to her son's wedding!

 ii. Triangulation—this is the unhealthy kind. As Crittenden points out in her trainings, healthy systems triangulate too, as in mother, father, child, with the child as the focus of the parents, but with equal focus on their partnership. The unhealthy kind is typically done in the manner described in the Karpman Drama Triangle,[17] where we find the Victim, the Oppressor, and the Rescuer.

iii. Spousification—this one is really bad: it's where the child is made into a surrogate spouse for the needy adult. This is done by the immature parent who is incapable of a fully adult romantic relationship with an age-appropriate partner and so makes the child into a lover. In all cases this is done for the gratification of the parent, not the good of the child. It is what is also known as 'emotional incest.' It is also identified as 'seductive parenting' in the book, *Development of the Person*.[18] Obviously, this would include sexual abuse as well. Such spousification is also likely to prompt resentment towards the child from the other parent and from other siblings who perceive the inappropriate elevation of the spousified child and irrationally blame the child for causing it. It's another one that I can personally attest to. Although the references cited are to seductive behaviour with toddlers, this pattern may extend throughout the child's life into adulthood.

6. Role Reversal—this goes beyond elevating the child to adult status (or demoting the parent to child status) and actually elevates the child to caregiving status *for* the parent rather than with the parent. This is reserved for children who have a parent strongly into the C4, feigned helpless strategy, or the depressed A strategy where the parent lacks the capacity to be responsive to their own needs, much less the child's.

7. Neglect—There are many examples and types of neglect: physical needs may be neglected, emotional needs may be neglected, and psychological developmental needs may be neglected. This neglect may be due to a lack of ability, as in unable to pay for what is needed, not noticed by the parent by their own preoccupation with their own unmet needs, noticed but the parent unable to respond effectively, noticed but misunderstood by the parent, and worst of all, noticed and resented or punished. Either way, the child's needs are simply not met by the parent. That in itself is bad enough in its effect on the child's development. Often, however, the most devastating impact of neglect is that the child learns to neglect their own needs (the A strategy) or becomes excessively preoccupied with them (the C strategy.)

8. Performance—Performance is when the parents predicate their acceptance and love of the child on the child's performance in whatever the parents' preferred mode of performance may be. This creates difficulty in a number of ways. First of all, perfection is expected, and anything less is rejected. Since perfection is virtually impossible, this can lead to long-term depression and procrastination, which is the opposite of 'perfection.' Second, it robs life of enjoyment. If expectations are set, then achieving them simply avoids a negative. (If preferences are set, then if they are met, we are pleased, but if not then it's no big deal.) Third, because parental approval is contingent on exceptional performance, the child grows up to become a 'human doing' rather than a 'human being.' They don't feel good about themselves in their own right, but rather in their accomplishments.

9. Deception—This is when the parents actively deceive the child. This deception can take many forms and is typically used to manipulate the child. When accompanied by actual danger it is especially damaging. It is often used in conjunction with these other constructs. For example, one parent may deceive the child regarding the other parent as a part of triangulation or as an aspect of sexual boundary violations. Often it involves the parent colluding with the child to deceive others. For example, I once had a parent who was complaining about his son deceiving him. He was very down on the son for not being truthful. Then, later in the session, he told me he was taking this same son to Florida for holiday the next week. When I enquired how he was going to manage that since school was in session, he said that he had instructed the son to lie to the teacher about the reason for his absence! He seemed blissfully unaware of any incongruence.

10. Sexuality—When sexuality is a construct, it has become overemphasized and is often intruded into the interview early and inappropriately and may be pervasive. It is often associated with the A5, Compulsive Promiscuity classification, or the C6, Seductive classification. It is generally associated with inappropriate sexualization of the child by the parent as a part of another construct, such as spousification or triangulation.

Dispositional Representations and Their Integration

Crittenden and Landini state that 'representation creates a disposition to act.' A dispositional representation is a *disposition* based on a *representation*. We all have 'inherent qualities of mind and character.' We then utilize these qualities of mind and character, such as thinking emotionally or logically, being generous and warm hearted or cold and stingy, in forming a representation of people and events. If I see a look on your face, I might interpret it as you needing a smile, a hug, and a reassuring or comforting message, or conversely, as you being a threat against which I must be prepared to defend myself. It could be the same look in each case, and you could be the same person. The only difference is *my* 'dispositional representation' or DR.

What determines my DR in regard to the look on your face? Why, my past experiences, of course, and the mental map of the world that I have stored there, and your place in that mental map of the world. As Crittenden puts it, 'The only information we have is about the past. The only information we need is about the future.' In other words, we are left to make our decisions on what to do in the future based on what we have experienced in the past. Most of the time, we can do this reliably without too much thought or conflict. But sometimes we make the wrong choice because our 'dispositional representation'—our default strategy—is out of sync with reality.

In determining the DR they refer to 'procedural, imaged, semantic, connotative and episodic dispositional representations and their integration.' These additional elements are the memory systems on which we rely for retrieving and processing information. We will take them in order.

Implicit Memory

First is the general category of implicit memory systems. Implicit means that they are operating below the surface and of which we are unable to be aware, except in some instances where we can access the information of how we formed the skill. There are two:

1. Procedural—Procedural memory refers to how we do things. Things like walking, talking, riding a bicycle, driving a car, or rolling a kayak. And it's not just performance type things, although performance is an aspect of it. It also includes how we process information. In other words, we have learned a *procedure* for *processing* information. They break this down into three parts:

a. How discourse is managed—that is, how I, the interviewee, manage to communicate with you, the interviewer. (That's a good example of role reversal, by the way.) For example, I might beat around the bush and never get to the point. Or, I might be blunt and direct, or cutting and sarcastic, or open and straightforward.

b. Spontaneous expression of affect—this refers to whether or not emotion is exhibited in response to the interview questions. For example, a sharp intake of breath followed by, 'Oh my God!' with a look of fear or surprise on my face would be a spontaneous expression of affect.

c. Patterns of interactive behaviour with the interviewer—for example, if I persistently ask the interviewer for confirmation that I am right in my explanation of events, or I might persistently wander off topic.

These various aspects of *how* we answer will be clues to help understand *what* we answer.

2. Imaged memory—These are images contained in the unconscious mind. Many of us tend to think in visual images. Thus, we might say, 'I can see it now,' followed by a vivid description of the sunny garden we were in when we learned our father was dead. Or, if we are kinaesthetic, we might be describing being struck by a parent with the words, 'the short, sharp, shock of it,' complete with an involuntary drawing back and raising the hand, as if to ward off a blow. An auditory image is, 'And the door slammed.' 'I could smell the beer on his breath when he was abusing me,' is olfactory. The olfactory sense is very powerful and can access other memory systems. The smell of the dental office, for example. Another visual is, 'where the skeletons are' in an answer to the first question in the AAI. When we were discussing that answer in a session, she vehemently denied using that expression. Why would she? But I had the recording. She said it. The 'skeletons in the closet' is implied because the full expression is not used but rather alluded to. The phrase was available to her unconscious mind or implicit memory, when she was answering the question, but when we were discussing it later it was so deeply inaccessible to the *conscious* mind, or explicit memory, that she absolutely denied that she would have ever said it.

Explicit Memory

Next come explicit memory systems. These, because they are not 'buried' in the unconscious, are memory systems that require intentional and conscious access of information, to include a decision as to what or how much to share, although this will also obviously be controlled initially by the implicit memory systems. The explicit decision making comes on top of that. To put it another way, the implicit memory systems—the ones running below awareness—respond to the question by giving us a range of options for answering, presenting the most likely first. We then choose whether or not to give that answer, reject it and get the next one, and the next, if necessary, to include consciously—or explicitly—altering the information that we choose to provide to the interviewer. The first of these is semantic memory.

1. Semantic Memory—This is described as being general knowledge. For example, 'If I was a good boy, she would be loving and kind, but if I was bad, she could be angry.' This is a statement of contingencies that may or may not happen. As such, it retains a hypothetical quality. I am not actually stating that I was ever either good or bad, or that she was loving and kind or angry. You, the listener, are left to fill in the vacuum with your own images of those hypothetical events. Or I might say, 'We were a happy family, very normal.' This is my subjective impression only. It presumes that families are normally happy. Notice that it also conflates 'happy' and 'very' to give the listener the impression of 'very happy' without actually saying that. It gives us a general description without telling us anything specific.

2. Connotative Language—This is a memory system that is proposed by Crittenden and Landini, which they describe as 'the verbalized form of an implicit memory system, in this case imaged memory.' Thus, if a speaker says, 'Sometimes I would be punished,' that by itself is dry and contingent and does not evoke any particular feeling or imagery. It is semantic only. If, on the other hand, I said 'My Dad used to fly into a rage and slap me around. Whop! Upside my head! I can still hear my ears ring.' That is evocative.

3. Episodic Memory—These are memories of actual events that occurred in the past and that we can now recount in sufficient detail to give the listener—and ourselves—an accurate and fairly complete description of what happened. Or not. Episodes may be omitted, or hypothetical, if our semantic description of childhood is inconsistent

with what actually occurred. They may be incomplete when we want to win favour by omitting what we did to set events in motion. Or we may leave our audience hanging by getting to the climax but eliminating the denouement. Episodic memory can be quite intrusive when the episodes are emotionally charged or completely repressed by the unconscious mind when remembering them is too painful. Or both. Oftentimes, when memories are completely repressed *and* emotionally charged, the emotion breaks through when triggered by an unrelated and often innocuous event. Sometimes the repression is not complete. Oftentimes, traumatic events are evidenced by intrusive memory fragments, like a giant penis descending from the sky right above the persons head, disconnected, ambiguous, disconcerting, to say the least.

4. Source Memory—This is the last piece of the puzzle. It refers to being able to recall where information came from. Some studies have found, for example, that when extremely threatening events take place, memory is often distorted. This is often a difficulty with so-called eyewitness testimony in court cases, which is notoriously unreliable. Witnesses, even as adults, can become convinced that they saw something that they didn't see because it has been suggested to them by the police or the prosecution. I once represented a couple of guys charge with arson. They were big and little, like Mutt and Jeff in the cartoon. An eyewitness swore it was the big guy who had kicked in the door and set fire to the place. In fact, (according to my clients) it was the little guy who had actually done the deed while the big guy acted as lookout. Or another case where my client insisted to me, after hearing the witness' testimony, 'No man, it wasn't me with the sawed-off shotgun! It was my buddy. I had the .45!' In both cases the 'eyewitnesses' were, by the perpetrators admissions, quite wrong in their identification. I'm not sure what they thought I could do with that information! The point is, the 'eyewitnesses,' who had sworn to tell the truth, insisted that was what they had seen with their own eyes, when in fact it was what they had been convinced to believe by the police and the prosecutors.

In a more applicable manner, clients will often, when recalling events, state that they don't know how they remember an event: whether they actually remember it, or whether they think they remember it because they were told about it. Or they saw a picture of it. This becomes particularly important for events early in childhood, as children need to be helped to know where their information comes from. Children, as we know, think magically, so a child might say, 'I know because a fairy told me so. She whispered it in my ear.' This takes on even more importance when a parent actively deceives the child.

Reflective Integration
This is the last bit of dispositional representations: reflective integration. It is what Crittenden and Landini identify as 'working memory.' It is a process that relies on memory and putting disparate pieces of information together in a process that we call 'reflective,' meaning we become aware of what we are doing in our minds with the information that we have at our disposal. We will be looking at examples of this process a bit later. Right now, though, I will give you an example that you can enjoy at your earliest opportunity.

Consider the sunset. If you go to watch the sunset, perhaps in a beautiful setting, with someone you love, and the weather is nice, with those high, wispy, overhead clouds that light up the sky with gorgeous colours just as the sun is setting, then you feel a thrill in your heart and your spirit at the majesty of creation, and you can actually feel the movement of the sun as it sinks below the horizon.

Except, it isn't the 'sun setting' that you are seeing. That is an illusion. What you are seeing is the rotation of the earth that is carrying you along at roughly 1000 miles per hour *away from* the sun—1037.561 mph to be exact, if you are at the equator at the equinox, less as you move away from the equator into different latitudes, compensating for the tilt of your position on the earth towards or away from the sun for days other than an equinox, and also by the earth's orbiting of the sun. We won't even think about the sun's rotation relative to the galactic centre. You are going backwards at that speed as the sun is blocked from view by your position changing relative to it by the rotation of the earth.

Now, the two preceding paragraphs are written from, first, the affective perspective and, second, the cognitive perspective. We can reflect on the different perspectives and the meaning they produce in our minds. But now, what if we put them both together, the cognitive and the affective? We have both the glory of the colours of the sunset and the majestic spectacle of the darkening sky, plus the knowledge of the tremendous forces hurtling us through the cosmos on our journey to we know not where. Wow! Does that make your heart go pitter-patter or what?

Reflective integration is what we do when we put things together in a different way or confirm that what we have previously done is accurate, so far as we know. Or if it is not accurate, how can we make it more accurate. It is being able to think about our thinking and have feelings about our feelings. It's also having thoughts about our feelings and feelings about our thoughts. And when we do all those things, it's truly reflective. It allows us to create a more coherent narrative of our life story.

Discourse Markers

Here are the DMM-AAI discourse markers given by Crittenden and Landini[19]:

Discourse Marker	Strategy	Memory System	Subset
Non-transforming dysfluency	B	Procedural memory	Discourse
Appropriate non-verbal affect	B	Procedural memory	Expression of affect
Cooperative	B	Procedural memory	Rel. w/interviewer
Fresh and integrated images	B	Imaged memory	
Differentiated generalizations	B	Semantic memory	
Spontaneous, lively discourse	B	Connotative language	
Complete episodes	B	Episodic memory	
Credible evidence	B	Episodic memory	
Reflective functioning	B	Reflective integration	
Metacognition	B	Reflective integration	
Distancing discourse	A	Procedural memory	Discourse
Disparaging humour	A	Procedural memory	Expression of affect
Omitted true negative affect	A	Procedural memory	Expression of affect
False positive affect	A	Procedural memory	Expression of affect
Denied negative affect and physical pain	A	Procedural memory	Expression of affect
Neutral	A	Procedural memory	Rel. w/interviewer
Analytical	A	Procedural memory	Rel. w/interviewer
Deference to others	A	Procedural memory	Rel. w/interviewer
Omitted images	A	Imaged memory	
Displaced images	A	Imaged memory	
Unconnected images	A	Imaged memory	
Delusionally protective images	A	Imaged memory	
Delusionally punitive images	A	Imaged memory	

(*continued*)

(continued)

Discourse Marker	Strategy	Memory System	Subset
Idealization	A	Semantic memory	
Exoneration	A	Semantic memory	
Self-responsibility	A	Semantic memory	
Misattribution of intent	A	Semantic memory	
Non-agency	A	Semantic memory	
Artificial language	A	Connotative language	
Cut-off or opposite episodes	A	Episodic memory	
Lack of recall of positive episodes	A	Episodic memory	
Displaced episodes and negative affect	A	Episodic memory	
Parental perspective	A	Episodic memory	
Distorted guilt	A	Episodic memory	
Delusional idealization	A	Episodic memory	
External reference	A	Episodic memory	
Omitted integration	A	Reflective integration	
Platitudes	A	Reflective integration	
Failed metacognitions	A	Reflective integration	
Inconclusive metacognitions	A	Reflective integration	
Involving discourse	C	Procedural memory	Discourse
Involving anger	C	Procedural memory	Discourse
Involving fear	C	Procedural memory	Discourse
Disarming affect	C	Procedural memory	Expression of affect
Mocking/Gotcha humour	C	Procedural memory	Expression of affect
Arousing non-verbal affect	C	Procedural memory	Expression of affect
Distorted positive affect	C	Procedural memory	Expression of affect
Cold or sadistically cruel affect	C	Procedural memory	Expression of affect
Involving	C	Procedural memory	Rel. w/interviewer
Confronting/collusive	C	Procedural memory	Rel. w/interviewer
Appealing/submissive	C	Procedural memory	Rel. w/interviewer
Parrying	C	Procedural memory	Rel. w/interviewer
Seductive	C	Procedural memory	Rel. w/interviewer
Intimidating/spooky	C	Procedural memory	Rel. w/interviewer
Intense images	C	Imaged memory	
Animated images (anger, fear, desire for comfort)	C	Imaged memory	
Generalized images	C	Imaged memory	
Delusionally threatening images	C	Imaged memory	
Passive semantic thought	C	Semantic memory	

(continued)

(continued)

Discourse Marker	Strategy	Memory System	Subset
Idealized expectations about the future	C	Semantic memory	
Reductionist blaming thought	C	Semantic memory	
Derogation	C	Semantic memory	
Person-defined negative meaning	C	Semantic memory	
Misattribution of causality	C	Semantic memory	
False cognition	C	Semantic memory	
Denial of responsibility	C	Semantic memory	
Evocative language	C	Connotative language	
Blurred or circular episodes	C	Episodic memory	
Lack of a negative episode	C	Episodic memory	
Fragmented episode	C	Episodic memory	
Negative episode but no harm to self	C	Episodic memory	
Triangulated episodes	C	Episodic memory	
False innocence/blame	C	Episodic memory	
Delusional revenge	C	Episodic memory	
Omitted integration	C	Reflective integration	
Pseudo-reflections	C	Reflective integration	
Rationalization	C	Reflective integration	
Skilful misleading	C	Reflective integration	
78 discourse markers: 10 B; 30 A; 37 C			

There are 78: 10 for the B strategy, evincing the simplicity and straight-forwardness of the B information processing. A comes second with 29, almost three times the number for B. C gets the prize for the most at 37 reflecting the complicated nature of the C strategy. I suppose that is due to the C strategy being somewhat in the middle: they vacillate between fear and the desire for comfort versus anger and revenge.

We will not discuss each of these discourse markers. Some are probably self-explanatory, the simplest being the first, 'non-transforming dysfluency.' For example, if someone asks a question, I might begin with, 'Erm …' while I gather my thoughts. On the other hand, 'Erm …, well, it's fair to say … that is … where my father is concerned … well, anyone, really, you could say that.' Now we are getting into some serious dysfluency. It still might not mean that much. No single discourse marker is going to be dispositive. You will be looking for patterns in the discourse, and how the discourse marker is being used. In other words, what is the meaning? What is its function? This is where the relationship with the interviewer is critical. How is the interviewee trying to influence the interviewer? These are all things that we look at when processing the interview with the client.

WHAT IF YOU AREN'T TRAINED?

As I hope I have adequately described, I began developing this method of working before getting any training in using the AAI. My unconscious incompetence was breached when I began to learn about attachment concepts. Simply explaining these basic concepts to clients enabled them to self-identify and create new meanings for themselves from the information shared. I quickly became aware of my conscious incompetence even as I applied what I thought that I knew of it. This fairly quickly led to my realization that I needed to aspire to achieving conscious competence.

I began using the AAI after I had my first week of training with Crittenden. That gave me the AAI, directions for administering it, and the rudiments of coding. I strongly urge you to get training as soon as possible. The basic course is 3 weeks will give you a thorough introduction to the method. You will administered the AAI to others and have your own AAI done. You will then be able to use the AAI with your clients. After all, if you have a very useful tool, why not use it? That it might not be of as much use to you and your client now as it will be later on is no reason not to use your knowledge now. Knowledge is always incomplete and expanding.

Simply understanding attachment theory and the three basic strategy categories, A, B, and C, can be very useful to you and your clients, as they were to mine early on. I did not have success using attachment concepts *after* I got training. I had success with Attachment Centred Therapy *before* I had any formal training, and that is what convinced me that it would be worth the time and money to get the training. Actually, I became convinced that it was *essential* that I get the training if I was going to hold myself out as dealing with attachment issues. And in my experience, most of the issues we encounter as therapists are attachment related.

You also have the option to get someone else to administer the AAI, someone to code it and provide you with a report, and someone to supervise you as you work through the AAI with the client. The more people there are who are trained to do these things, the more resources there will be available. Training will also put you in touch with others who are qualified to code the AAI. This will be a valuable resource, especially when you encounter transcripts that are challenging to code.

I also suggest that you be wary of getting your information about attachment off the internet. There is a lot of misunderstanding out there, as the references I have given prove, at least, to my satisfaction. To state this as 'proof' is strong stuff. So let me just ask a few questions. Do you consider someone who is writing an article or a book critical of attachment theory to be knowledgeable enough about the topic to be credible if they are unaware of the existence of two differing models of attachment? Do you, as a scientist, regard the *assumption* that a mother will somehow 'transmit' her attachment strategy to her infant child to be valid and supported by the evidence of your own observations? After reading this article,[20] written by the creators and defenders of the D category: (a) do you think the D classification does more harm than good? (b) Do you think the authors are accepting or evading responsibility for having created a misleading classification that has caused great injustice in deciding child welfare issues, essentially blaming the users of their product?

We, as practicing professionals, have a duty to seek out the best information possible for helping our clients. Getting trained is up to you. So, I am working both sides of the street here. On the one hand, don't be afraid to discuss attachment concepts and implications with your clients, but be careful about what you think you know. That is one of the reasons it has taken me 20 years to write this book. I do ask myself, do I really know what I am talking about? And, I still don't know the answer to that question.

What I do know is that getting the training in the DMM-AAI and using ACT has transformed how I do therapy. And no, I don't base that on my own subjective impressions, although they do align with that belief. Rather, it is based on what my clients report to me and what I observe in their behaviour. Theory must follow observation. Never the other way 'round.

NOTES

1. Fraley, R. C., Heffernan, M. E., Vicary, A. M., & Brumbaugh, C. C. (2011). The experiences in close relationships—Relationship Structures Questionnaire: A method for assessing attachment orientations across relationships. *Psychological assessment, 23*(3), 615.
2. Holmes, J. (2014). *The search for the secure base: Attachment theory and psychotherapy.* Routledge.
3. Ainsworth, M. D. S., Blehar, M. C., Waters, E., & Wall, S. (1978). Strange situation procedure. *Clinical Child Psychology and Psychiatry.*
4. Granqvist, P., Sroufe, L. A., Dozier, M., Hesse, E., Steele, M., van IJzendoorn, M., … & Duschinsky, R. (2017). Disorganized attachment in infancy: A review of the phenomenon and its implications for clinicians and policy-makers. *Attachment & human development, 19*(6), 534–558. This article does not repudiate the 'D' classification. To the contrary, it gaslights in that it places all the blame squarely on the naïve users of this flawed idea.
5. Meins, E. (2017). The predictive power of attachment. *Psychologist, 30*(1), 21–24.
6. Keller, H. (2021). *The myth of attachment theory: A critical understanding for multicultural societies.* Routledge.
7. Used with permission of Patricia M. Crittenden: https://familyrelationsinstitute.org/dmm-model/.
8. Bejan, A. (2019). *Freedom and evolution: hierarchy in nature, society and science.* Springer Nature.
9. https://familyrelationsinstitute.org/trainer/patricia-crittenden/.
10. Bakermans-Kranenburg, M. J., & Van IJzendoorn, M. H. (1993). A psychometric study of the Adult Attachment Interview: Reliability and discriminant validity. *Developmental psychology, 29*(5), 870.
11. To learn about trainings, when and where they will be held, visit https://familyrelationsinstitute.org/course/adult-attachment-interview-online-training-by-zoom/.
12. Crittenden, P. M., & Landini, A. (2011). *Assessing adult attachment: A dynamic-maturational approach to discourse analysis.* WW Norton & Company.
13. Grice, H. P. (1975). Logic and conversation. In *Speech acts* (pp. 41–58). Brill.
14. Asada, K., Itakura, S., Okanda, M., Moriguchi, Y., Yokawa, K., Kumagaya, S., … & Konishi, Y. (2022). Understanding of the Gricean maxims in children with autism spectrum disorder: Implications for pragmatic language development. *Journal of Neurolinguistics, 63*, 101,085. Wahyunianto, D., Djatmika, D., & Purnanto, D. (2020). Grice's Cooperative Principles Violation in the Communication of Children with Autism. *Sosiohumaniora, 22*(1), 36–45.

15. Crittenden, P. M., & Landini, A. (2011). *Assessing adult attachment: A dynamic-maturational approach to discourse analysis.* WW Norton & Company.
16. Ibid., p. 70.
17. https://karpmandramatriangle.com/.
18. Sroufe, L. A., Egeland, B., Carlson, E. A., & Collins, W. A. (2009). *The development of the person: The Minnesota study of risk and adaptation from birth to adulthood.* Guilford Press. Sroufe, L. A., & Ward, M. J. (1980). Seductive behavior of mothers of toddlers: Occurrence, correlates, and family origins. *Child Development*, 1222–1229.
19. Crittenden, P. M., & Landini, A. (2011). *Assessing adult attachment: A dynamic-maturational approach to discourse analysis.* WW Norton & Company.
20. Granqvist, P., Sroufe, L. A., Dozier, M., Hesse, E., Steele, M., van Ijzendoorn, M., … & Duschinsky, R. (2017). Disorganized attachment in infancy: A review of the phenomenon and its implications for clinicians and policy-makers. *Attachment & human development, 19*(6), 534–558.

CHAPTER 4

Working with the Transcript

The preceding chapters give an overview from a theoretical perspective: a road map, if you will. This chapter discusses the real work, where the rubber meets the road: working through the transcript with the client. My purpose in devising this method was to help my clients in the best way possible. The initial meeting is to establish rapport, to determine the client's needs, to discuss with the client how ACT can meet those needs, and to form an agreement to go ahead with the interview. Because it does represent a significant investment of time and money, the client needs to understand what they are getting into. I explain how I work back and forth by using the AAI to understand the challenges they are facing and what they want to achieve in therapy, and then to understand the choices they are making in their lives and how that informs what we are discovering in the AAI. Sessions will often involve both the talk therapy of discussing events in their lives and reading segments of the AAI. Sometimes it will be one or the other, but always being mindful of the other aspect.

In order to keep track of where we are, I draw a line under the section of the AAI that we have covered for that session, put the notation, 'stopped here' with the date. Then on the front page of the transcript, I note the page number and the date and put a box around it. That way I can quickly go to where we left off in the previous session. Sometimes I think it important to return to a section that we discussed in the previous AAI session. In that case I put a box around the relevant section. I have spent several

C. Shults, *Attachment Centred Therapy*, Palgrave Texts in Counselling and Psychotherapy, https://doi.org/10.1007/978-3-031-60851-3_4

sessions on a single sentence. That is a part of the power of the method: we can dig deeper and deeper into the layers of meaning and experience, especially when we are working with something that the client can change or observe in their life and relationships.

When I first began using this method, I coded the transcript in its entirety just the way I was taught and came up with a tentative classification. I charged extra for that because of the time that it took. Then one day a client asked me if I would do the coding in the session, as he didn't want to pay the extra charge for it to be coded in advance. I thought it over and told him that I was willing to give that a try. However, I made clear that was not the way that I was trained to do it, and that our use of time in the sessions would be less efficient since I would not have prepared the transcript in advance and would have to spend time finding the discourse markers. I also would not have taken the time to have thought about it before hand, and so it might take longer to work out what the discourse markers might mean. They form patterns, after all, and those patterns are what determine the classification.

He replied that he didn't mind if it cost more long term or if it took longer, so I gave it a try. To my pleasant surprise, it seemed to work better that way. Even though it did take longer than it would have for me to simply go over it with him having coded it in advance, going through it together seemed to add a dimension of teamwork, exploration, and discovery. As I read through the transcript, and came to each discourse marker I would explain it to him and give my idea of what it might mean and how it might be functioning in this context. Sometimes I even read sections from Crittenden's website or *Assessing Adult Attachment*.[1] He could then give me his insight into what he thought it might mean. Not only did he have the memory of the original event, he also had the memory of what he thought or felt as he answered the question on the AAI, and what he thought and felt as we were reading it together.

After that positive experience, I began to give clients the option of me coding in advance or doing it as we go. Eventually, I became convinced that coding the transcript as we go through it together adds a richness to the experience. Not only do we explore the meaning of the transcript together, it also gives us the opportunity to form a team for exploration.

It is perhaps natural to wonder if sharing the discourse markers, for example, reductionist blaming thought, or person-defined negative meaning, might be off-putting to the clients. I have not found it to be so. To the contrary, clients seem to like learning about themselves. When I was starting out in the treatment centre, our staff psychologist routinely did psychometric testing. The MMPI (Minnesota Multiphasic Personality Inventory) was standard and patients would typically enquire about the results. We were admonished not to tell them. The attitude was one of secrecy: we, the staff, could know what the patient's results were on their psychological testing, but they couldn't. As a lawyer, this struck me as unfair and inappropriate. Being a bit of a contrarian and wanting to know if the accepted wisdom was really wise, I decided to test the theory.

What I learned was that clients were eager to know what their psychological testing said about them. They wanted to know what the different scales meant. I would explain to them. Sometimes they disagreed with the findings. I stressed that this was not gospel and the results were not infallible. Rather, they needed to think of it as being the test's interpretation of what they had told the test, as interpreted by the psychologist. I also stressed that this test result was in the context of being in a treatment centre for the use of mind altering chemicals that had created a pattern of addictively disordered behaviour.

What I found was that the patients would actively use this information in self-correcting. I find the same effect, only more so, with the DMM-AAI and ACT. Initially, clients will probably experience the 'shock of recognition' effect. You will, too, when you read your own part of the interview and recognize your own dysfluency, violations of Grice's Maxims, etc.

The Shock of Recognition

We experience this effect when we see or experience ourselves as others do. It might happen when you are walking down the street and unexpectedly see yourself reflected in a shop window. In my childhood it was hearing myself on a tape recorder and later seeing myself in a home movie. I was shocked in both instances, because the reality of how I looked and sounded, objectively, was very different from the subjective impression that I had of myself.

Clients will experience this 'shock of recognition' as they learn about themselves . Now, the nice thing about this 'shock of recognition' is that, once you get used to it—'it' being the thing that shocks you—it isn't that bad at all. We can learn to use the process of getting feedback in order to improve ourselves, and from that improved position make further improvements.

Many clients are embarrassed when they hear their dysfluent speech read back to them. I quickly reassure them, explain about the 'shock of recognition' effect, and let them know that I am often embarrassed by my own stumbling around, saying stupid things, and making mistakes of one sort or another. *It's okay!* We're only human, after all, and far from perfect. Typically, it doesn't take long for clients to accept their discourse as it is and as a faithful recording of what they said and how they said it. They can also use it as a benchmark for change.

The further shock of recognition is to be able to see how they process information and particularly the distortions of it. Clients can pretty quickly begin to understand, but it takes longer to change. Even in therapy sessions, clients become lost in their own information-processing errors. This is not 'resistance.' This is a clue to further impediments to information processing, and those are the unconscious mind defences against difficult information. What Crittenden refers to as 'the unknowable, the unspeakable, the unthinkable.'

Those 'uns' are what we are wanting to know about, speak about, and think about. And we want to do it in a balanced way. This is where it gets really exciting. As this information is accessed, we have the opportunity to create the narrative that will take us towards B3. As these matters have not been previously 'rehearsed' in the mind, we have the opportunity to programme the narrative in a more balanced way.

As clients reintegrate information that was previously denied, whether factual or emotional, they have to reintegrate those aspects of personality that were rejected and hidden in order to adapt to their attachment figures. Typically, this denied information will be with regard to losses. These are very real losses that need to be resolved in order for their life story to be more complete and more coherent.

This replicates the attachment experience with a caregiver even more so than having coded it in advance, I believe. Coding in advance seems to imply that I am 'the expert' and I am going to come up with a 'diagnosis' and then deliver the cure. Working through together makes it teamwork where we both contribute equally.

Another advantage is when there are ambiguous parts of the transcript. For example, answering a question with a question. This impacts the relationship with the interviewer. It could mean different things in context. A client might ask, in response to the first question asking about their family during their childhood years, 'What, you mean the early years?' This question could be part of an A, B, or C strategy. It could be part of an A4 strategy where the motivation is to make sure they comply accurately with the request. However, it could be a B strategy question, also wanting to make sure they are complying with the request. Or it could be a C strategy question that is somewhat challenging to the request, as in questioning what childhood could possibly have to do with today.

No individual discourse marker is going to be determinative of anything. The discourse markers create a pattern, and it is this pattern that gives us an understanding of what the transcript is conveying. Like the individual pixels that go to make a picture, these discourse markers create the overall 'picture' or attachment strategy. However, an individual discourse marker within an overall transcript can provide the key to solving the puzzle.

EDUCATION

The educational process works both ways. I am gaining information about the client. The client is gaining information about the AAI, discourse markers, and themselves. For example, in going through a transcript for the first time with a fairly new client, I noticed that she used a lot of always/never type of language. I pointed this out to her, with the caveat that we were just beginning with the transcript, that we humans often over generalize, and that it might not be important, but there it is.

'Oh no,' she replied. 'It is a big deal. My boyfriend complains about it *all the time!*'

Each discourse marker is explained and discussed as each appears and the client is educated about attachment ideas and principles. Eventually, you will also be able to identify the discourse markers in real time as clients make errors of information processing, or reorganize, during the session. This is an ideal time to intervene by pointing out the discourse marker in real time. Relate these to the ones found in the transcript and then correct the error. The error, once corrected, will lead to a new feeling state or a new insight, or both. Continue to do this. Eventually, the client will catch themselves making the error and will spontaneously correct it.

Also, please remember what I mean by 'error.' It is anything less than optimal information processing. This is another advantage of going through it with the client: the client may be able to answer the question immediately as to what this particular discourse marker means in the context of the transcript. Here is an example.

THE LONG KISS GOODNIGHT

I had recently completed a week of Crittenden's DMM-AAI training and I had thought, as we worked through the transcripts, that she was putting too much emphasis on tiny things in the transcript. However, as I was going through a transcript with a client, I came upon something that changed my mind completely and helped me to realize the power of the DMM-AAI.

There was a pause in a client's description of what happened when she went to bed at night. She was telling about her father putting her to bed and giving her a kiss every night. A lovely story. But there was a pause where there ought not to have been a pause: 'and then he would give me a ... a kiss goodnight.'

As I was going through the transcript with the client, I wondered aloud what the pause meant, while giving the caveat that it might not mean anything or that she might not remember. 'Oh no,' she replied, 'I remember exactly. I was trying to decide whether or not to tell you that, one night, he had kissed me in a way that wasn't a good night kiss.'

Whoa! The implication was obvious. The difficulty for the client appeared to be that the information she had paused briefly over was inconsistent with the idealized image she had constructed of her father. This was in contrast to her cold and disciplinarian mother, who was also cold and disciplinarian towards dad, in the client's telling. Hence the conflict, hence the pause.

That was the clue that, when wondered about openly with the client, led to the revelation of information that she had previously censored, which then, in my understanding, suddenly caused the pieces—the individual discourse markers—to fall into place in understanding the client's experience. We were able to reconstruct her history in a different, more coherent way that explained her present relationship difficulties.

For example, an episode with a sled in the snow had been related for the word, 'protective.' She and dad were sledding. The sled had gone swiftly downhill towards a stone fence, and dad had extended his feet beyond where the client was sitting in order to break the force of the collision. But ...

In the first place, dad was the one who had sent them down the hill towards the stone wall. We could code this episode as a 'delusionally protective image.' This is where the attachment figure does protect the child, but from a danger that the attachment figure has created. Second, as we reviewed the transcript with this new information, in response to my questioning dad being 'protective,' she volunteered the information that, indeed, after breaking the force of the collision with the stone wall, dad got off the sled and walked away, leaving her there by herself. This is a lack of comfort. We also reinterpreted much of their interactions as triangulation with mom. So the demonizing of mom and the idealizing of dad were interpreted to be 'reductionist blaming thought' and 'delusional idealization.' This leads me to a working hypothesis of an A/C strategy. A/C strategies often occur when the client, as here, has to adapt to a C strategy, mom's, and an A strategy, dad's. This then leads to sociopathic type behaviours such as cheating on one's partner, which is what had brought this client to therapy. And her partner was female while her cheating was with males.

In another example, there was this exchange in the interview:

> **And then finally was lazy if you have got an example of that?**
> Yeah so it was, it's basically just the fact that she never did anything really so throughout her life when I was alive erm she went through large periods of depression and inactivity she was **mm** unemployed and yeah just, not there and I remember times where for instance she, she would say like I really want you home so that we can spend time together but in that time she wouldn't do anything with me she would just watch TV **really** and, yeah that was her idea of us spending time together was us watching TV together and that's what I meant by lazy like she never tried to do anything, and yeah.
> **And did you watch TV together?**
> Well, she would watch TV. I would often read at the same time, but I would hide the book so that she thought I was   paying attention.
> **Okay—if she saw the book what would she do?**
> Probably throw it at me.
> **Mm, throw it at you?**
> Yeah.

There is a lot in this brief segment. First, it has a hypothetical, 'if … then …' quality: *if* she saw the book, *then* she would *probably* throw it at me. I explained this to Rebecca, my client, and then inquired if that had actually happened. Yes, she replied. How many times, I asked. Only once, she said. Oh really? I said. And then I enquired about the obvious discrepancy: if you had the book and was reading it, how did she throw it at you? I confess I thought that it would be mom snatching the book from her hand and throwing it at her. It was worse than that.

'Well,' she replied, 'she saw that I was reading something and she asked what it was. I told her it was a book. She wanted to know what kind of book so I told her and she asked me if she could see it. I told her yes and gave it to her. I was excited that she was interested in what I was reading and I thought that she might want to talk about it. But instead, she looked at it for a moment, and then she flew into a rage and threw it at me.'

I asked how old she was. Seven, she said.

In my opinion, whether to code the AAI in advance or not is optional. The advantage of coding it in advance is that you have already identified some of the discourse markers and have an idea of what they mean so that we can save time—and therefore money—in the therapy sessions. This is also informed by the fact that I was the interviewer, and so I have heard the client's AAI spoken and know their history and something of their affect and discourse markers when I begin coding. In the event that one is working with a client using the AAI without administering it, then of course one must read it first in order to have the proper context. It is also possible to have the transcript coded by someone else.

However one gets to it, we then start through the transcript together for the first time. In this first meeting, I go very slowly. That is because I am educating the client as to the possible meanings of the discourse markers as we go along. Education is one of the most important aspects of psychotherapy.

THE DILAPIDATED HOUSE

Following is an excerpt from a therapy session with a client. It is heavily edited to save time and space and to emphasize the point: using discourse markers in order to illuminate history. The therapy session is indented. When I am reading from the transcript, that will be double indented. My speech is in **bold**. Hers is in regular. My commentary will be in brackets. I will follow that format throughout the rest of the book.

She is fairly new in therapy at this point, as I give the interview as soon as I can in our work together because that is the way the client is going to get the most out of therapy. I begin by asking her what she wants to work on today, as I want to give the client control of the agenda:

> [Session:]
> Yeah I would like to have a look at the attachment interview.
> **Okay**

Could we erm, could we make a start on that?

We certainly can:

> **[Transcript:]**
> **Okay, orient me to your childhood family, erm who was in your family etc,**

you say:

> Okay, err so I was born in [name], mm we lived in a small village dash town called [name]. Mm, I lived with my mum and my dad and my younger sister, Yvonne. Err the other significant person in my life, was my, my nanna, my grandma who lived um very near to us in [name]. Mm, my dad was self-employed and owned mm two stores which were [deleted]. mm and he worked in those and um my mum erm helped him err with that and ran the house and looked after us.

Now that's all very concise. It's very appropriate. Err, it answers the question in all respects so that would get a B, or balanced, code. In other words, if the whole transcript was like that, we would say secure attachment. No unresolved problems from the past…

mm

…except (chuckle) here is where it gets slightly dysfluent. Have we talked about what a dysfluency is?

No.

Dysfluency is like, if I'm trying to explain dysfluency, and I start going: erm, um let's see err well you know dys … err dys … Dysfluency is what I just demonstrated there in my speech. It's like, 'Well, something is going on here.' Now *that* I was consciously doing just to, as an illustration. The one I *just* did when I said, 'just to, as an illustration,' was unintentional, and it is something that we all do to a certain extent, if you see what I mean?

Yeah.

And we are normally not used to our language or speech being put under the, the, (chuckling) well, microscope. Sometimes people find that a bit creepy or what I call it the shock of recognition. Sometimes, when you are getting an objective—like when you see yourself err in a picture or especially a video, you know and you see yourself for the first time. Sometimes the shock is like, 'What, that's me?!' You know, that image out there?

Yeah.

Or the sound of my voice. I recognise it's me but it's not the me that I have conceived of in my mind.

Yeah.

So back to the point: what am I finding here? So:

[The businesses are described] mm and he worked in those and um my mum um helped him um with that and ran the home and looked after us.
So, there is just a little bit of extra dysfluency around mum, working in the store that may or not be important, okay?
Yeah.
You say:
Yes, so he was a businessman and erm, mm invested in erm, property a little bit and the shops and that was basically what he did.
I am suspecting there is something about the business that's going on, maybe not. You know maybe I'm just noticing something unusual about it. And then your mom.   I say:
You said she helped him in the store is that right?
Yeah, my mom helped him and we lived in a house in [name]. We lived in the same house until um I was twelve years old, and then we moved to a house literally err less than a third of a mile away. It was a much bigger, err, older house, err quite grand if you like. Mm it was dilapidated, so we moved, we moved there when I was twelve.
Now err, this is the use of the word 'so' and this may seem to be going really slowly and, 'I am not getting a lot out of it right now…'
I, I am just taking it all on board Charley.
Yeah, because we are building a knowledge base right now, and I am not going to try to teach you everything about attachment or how to code transcripts but I do want to explain what's relevant.   Now the word 'so,' is sometimes a causation statement. Okay?   Erm: 'He wanted to get something to drink so he popped into the corner store to buy it.' So, 'so' (therefore) wanting to get a drink motivated him to do that. Causation. So here it's,
It was dilapidated so we moved, we moved there when I was twelve.
'So' in that sense it could mean, 'Because it was dilapidated we moved there.' do you see what I mean?
mm, mm
Which might be true because people sometimes move into dilapidated-houses in order to fix them up and sell them?
Yeah, they moved into the house. My parents wanted to have err this house, it was err, historically interesting, it had a very large garden and grounds around it so they liked the whole erm, they liked the whole, that, the whole house and it's grounds and that's what they wanted so they wanted to be there because it was a beautiful house even though it was dilapidated. They could see a lot of potential.
Yeah and you just used so again: 'therefore they moved there.' [Next we cover the questions about her grandparents which leads to:]

And my nanna I was incredibly close to,

So, okay. That is going to be important

and she was a big mm, she would, she was—very—I was,

There again we get dysfluency. is it …? We don't know why, it's just, there it is. I will continue to wonder why, but I—I the question in my mind now—and I am thinking real time, reflecting—could this have to do with, could it be connected to the dysfluency when you were talking about mom helping out in the stores and so on? I don't know. *We* don't know. if you have an idea you are welcome to say cause I will voice my wonderings, my musings out loud, and quite often that triggers people to give hugely important information. You just never know.

So this is an exploration err, the two of us, teamwork, I—I purport to know something about what these discourse markers represent, and you know the facts, the information that you have got stored in your mind, some of which will be distorted or repressed.

mm

And that's what we are looking for also.

mm

Erm, I was very close to her, she was always there for me and she always did things with us as a family, so yeah, had a lovely relationship with her,

Now we got our first big discourse marker: you left out the word 'I,' okay? This is the first time you have done it but believe it or not that is a significant discourse marker.

Okay

When we leave out the personal pronouns such as 'I,' 'we,' 'us,' again we don't know if it means anything or not, if it's part of a pattern because we don't have enough examples to have a pattern yet. Leaving out 'I' is indicative of an avoidant strategy. Erm, so we will see.

Do you know your mom's birth order?

She is an only child.

is she?

Yes so my mom is an only child. both of my, both set of grandparents were quite, mm, had quite humble beginnings and erm and for my maternal grandmother it was, a lot to have the child you know? It was, err, it was certainly something that was thought about,

I didn't pursue that at the time but I want to pursue it right now. Why was that a lot for her to think about?

My grandmother got pregnant with my mum and she wasn't married to my grandfather.

Okay.

And he was ten err I think he was almost ten years younger so in that era it caused a bit of a scandal.

Wait, who was younger?

My granddad was younger than my nanna so they, he erm, they had been seeing each other and she had got pregnant and they weren't married which in those days was frowned upon.

Well, absolutely. Erm, so how old was your grandmom when she had your mom? Do you know?

Err, I think she was in her mid-thirties which was old then.

Well, that's highly unusual.

Yeah.

Do you know why that was?

I don't know why it was that she, why she wasn't married by then. I don't know, erm and I—I—that I suppose is unusual, the fact that she wasn't married and she was in her, her thirties.

Cause how old, err, what year would she have been born?

Oh, goodness me.

Ballpark: just the era?

Erm, 19… err 1908 or something like that

1908 okay so that would have been … just before the start of World War I wasn't it? Erm okay. Erm, so they got married but your mum was the only child they had?

I think, I am not sure, but I think she might have had an abortion later on in her life

Oh really?

Yeah. I am not sure and it's something that I haven't talked about to my family.

Mm. So, there is often shame associated with that.

Yeah, I think so but also I think that I haven't wanted to—talk about something that could be painful.

Mm. Err, well I think you can eliminate the—the possibility there, because it's definitely going to be painful.

Mm

And I would say all the more reason to talk about it…

But it wasn't something … we had a conversation once in a café many years ago and she alluded to being pregnant and getting rid of the baby.

Oh, mm.

But I … think that I was so shocked I didn't quite take it in and I suppose I just then, just didn't talk about it.

Well that's what I mean, I mean err it's one of those difficult subjects.

By the way, there is no reason—I am certainly not intending to imply that one ought or should or must be ashamed. I think those are perfectly natural, normal things to happen in people's lives and usually when there is shame and condemnation about those it makes it harder to deal with, not easier. So, we don't know. We will see whether anything like that shows up err later.

Now we get to err the first, the earliest memory that you have as a child and this is often quite interesting because it gives us almost a thumbnail snapshot of what we are going to find in err in the transcript, you say:

> Err, one of the earliest memories is, mm, being in Portugal and my sister having had a finger trapped in a door and rushing to hospital, with her finger falling off.

Ooh, her finger falling off?

> Actually, it was actually a thumb and it was fine and everything was okay but I just remember that's one of my earliest memories. I was three.

She was younger by how much?

> She was two years younger.

So, she would have been one year old. Erm, and I say:

> **Tell me as much as you can remember about it.**
>
> I can just remember flashbacks of the, of the holiday, I can remember driving past orange and lemon trees and I can remember seeing the swimming pool and I remember a hotel bar and the door of the room where she got her finger trapped. Err, those are the things that I can remember.
>
> **So what do you remember about that? About her finger trapped in the door?**
>
> Just the screaming and the err.... Just the screaming really, and, err, not much more.
>
> **Okay. Err any images that go with it?**
>
> Just um err like a sort of plaster-cum-err-bandage that went over her thumb. I just remember that.
>
> **Okay. And you said her finger was falling off, but um,**
>
> It was, it was blood and it was the tip of her finger and she had to have it stitched back on.

Oh gosh, so a lot of mmm ... I said:

> **So she didn't lose her finger?**
>
> No, she didn't lose her finger. I am making it sound really gory and it's not as gory as I am saying at all (laughing).

Now that's interesting because this I'm going to label reflective functioning, and we really like reflective functioning, yeah? Reflective functioning is when you are saying, 'no she didn't lose a finger,' and you are commenting on your earlier comments. You say 'I am making it sound really gory and it's not as gory as I am saying at all,' and a chuckle. Okay? So number one, that's a recognition, well that's okay to do that because we ask for your memory, yeah? 'Tell me about what happened in that memory' and you told me,.

Mm.

And it's very likely that as a three year old that was the first time you had encountered something like that, okay?

Yeah.

And even though it was the tip of a finger or a thumb I can imagine that that would have been quite a shock to you...

Mm.

Yeah? and she had to have it sewn back on.

Mm.

So you are reflecting on: yeah when I tell it from my childhood perspective it was awful but you know looking back on it now it wasn't that, it wasn't like she was going to lose that finger, but I didn't know that as a child.

Mm, yeah.

So reflective functioning is good. Then:

> Describe your relationship with your mother as far back as you can remember?

You say:

> Err, she was always somebody that I could rely on, I called her Jennifer from being three, I didn't call her mom or mommy, I called her Jennifer and people used to say, 'Why do you call her Jennifer,' and I said, 'Well, because everybody else does so I am going to call her Jennifer, too.' Mm, occasionally I would call her mummy. But I liked calling her Jennifer. Err, she, err, she was an amazing cook when we were growing up. We had fantastic meals. The house was beautiful. So, she was into antiques and interior design and especially gardening. She had a lovely garden and she loved to spend time gardening. Mm, she used to help my dad with the business, err, and she used to work in the shop when, err, we moved house and money was tight. She set up a market garden business and things were really bad then financially for my parents and there was very little money so she kept us going by selling fruit and vegetables and flowers that we sold at the gate of the house and I remember as a child helping with that.

Err now was that before or after you moved into the err, big, dilapidated house?

Afterwards.

That's what I thought. So she would grow vegetables in the garden and flowers, erm and err, du du du du—'someone I could rely on,' okay. Erm what I am going to note here is that err, this interestingly this sounds like an A, avoidant type answer because there is not much about feelings in here. There are feelings expressed for example fantastic meals okay? We have a corner shop that serves fantastic meals. That doesn't tell us anything about the nature of the relationship, if you see what I mean?

Yeah.

Yeah. Erm, 'somebody that I could rely on' does erm. so there's a distancing quality to your relationship with mom which I find that surprising because overall err—I, I would have predicted that you were on the C side of the spectrum because err, of the, I suppose the degree of upset or err, the distress that I… observed you know when we were first interacting and you know these problems that were besetting you. Now, you can be a secure B3, you know, the gold standard of security, and be upset and distressed about events. So, anyway, I am just sharing some of my processing out loud as we speak, but based on this answer and the dropping out of the 'I' earlier I would say maybe there is some avoidance going on here, I am always happy to be wrong. I am always happy to change my mind and plus, it doesn't matter what strategy I think you are using. It's what you decide and what you choose for yourself that's important.

Mm.

My job is to help you do that, not to decide something and try to impose it on you.

Mm.

Does that make sense?

Yeah. Yeah.

Erm, okay, and I had already asked about moving into the other house, let me read this because I want to see what you are saying. You say:

> Yeah, we moved into the other house and it was huge, massive house um and as soon as we moved into the house um, um my dad became very fixated on the house, the building and err, he became obsessed with mm doing renovation to the house, but in a very strange order. For example he would spend, he spent a lot of money on the lawn behind the house, okay—and he spent a lot of money on the stables that were attached to the house. And we had no kitchen in the house.

Good lord! I mean, I am doing the exaggeration now!
Yeah. Yeah.
We had no … The walls were covered in mould and the wallpaper was hanging off and there were holes in the carpet and it was holes and damp, and then there was a big hole um from the front door to the, to the entry hall that we had to walk over a plank for a couple of years because he started digging it up and it hadn't, he hadn't fixed it. Um, it was, the house was a real state, mm, yeah, and my mom was just trying to manage doing this house, mm, and err yeah it was err, it was difficult. That was the start of some very difficult times.
This is a perfect place to stop. Because, err—yeah now err,—now we know what these discourse markers that were on the first page were about okay?
Mm.
Probably. **Again, I may make a statement that sounds absolutely definitive, but always remember: it's a hypothesis. But the odds are, in the first paragraph and um 'my mum erm helped him erm with that, and ran the home and looked after us,' that is probably presaging, that is a very good semantic description, an overall description of the history and it takes into account both the time prior to the move and the time after the move because that's why it's not completely dysfluent because when you moved in there err, in, and also it would explain the so, the 'so we moved, we moved there when I was twelve,' and it does sound as if your dad bought a fixer upper and it does sound that the 'so,' the 'because' that I mentioned on page one it is, it was causation. Dad wanted to move there so he could fix it up, and probably knowing what I know about such projects and such situations, mum had not realised what she was getting into, that it was going to be so much chaos and you had just said how important having a nice house was to her, yeah?**
Mm.
So now we have a real clash of values between mom and dad.
Mm.
Did they stay together or did they split up?
They divorced.
How old were you when they divorced?
Err they started divorcing when I was about fourteen, fifteen.
Okay, so the house broke the marriage?
Yeah, the house yeah definitely broke the marriage.
I say broke, I mean there may have been other dynamics at work?
Yeah. It was certainly err a factor.

It's really hard to understand some of the choices he made err but anyway I don't know that we have to. **Do you ever wonder about that yourself?**
Yeah, I often used to think, why on earth was he doing that or why was he, why was he, why was he spending money on something that we didn't need when we could have done with a kitchen, or we could have done with filling holes up in the floor. Why was he, why was he spending money on things that didn't seem logical.
They weren't logical and so—what we will be looking for, because I think those are legitimate questions and they can be important in terms of understanding parental motivation and therefore can help in resolution of any unresolved issues, and again the, the disfluency that we find is indicative of an unresolved issue, yeah?
You know Charley this feels so exhausting. Is this normal? I feel really, I feel very, very tired and I feel very—erm, I just feel very, very, err, heavy I don't quite know how to explain it.
I was going to suggest sad.
Yeah it think it's more, it's more than sadness. I feel exhausted. Yeah, a little bit sad I suppose, but the overwhelming for me is absolute exhaustion.
Well, when did this feeling of exhaustion set in?
What this morning—over this, over this when you were reading through these things, cause I felt a heaviness as you were … the more that you got into it, I started to feel heavier.
Of course.
And heavier.
Of course you did.
And more and more tired.
Because?
Erm, I suppose … sorry. I suppose I feel tired anyway. I feel … very drained, very burnt out in my life generally and hearing this, just feels really … it's just hard, actually to hear it, and you are not saying anything that's seemingly traumatic. It's just, I suppose I find it hard to think back to that time because I am finding it very—part of me just doesn't want to do that.
Yeah.
Part of me wants to just brush it under the rug and pretend that it's not happened or happening or it's not even part of my being.
And that's the denial. That's the first phase in the grieving process.
Is it?
It is. Have we talked about the grieving process?
Yeah.
The denial, anger, blaming and bargaining, sadness and depression and then finally acceptance?

Mm.

Erm, it's a challenge Claudia,

Mm.

And it's just like what I think I was saying to you earlier in this session: people often resist getting in touch with unresolved stuff from the past because they think, 'Oh, that will be painful. I don't want to have to deal with that.'

Yeah, that's true.

I am willing to hear any exceptions if they come along, but, it's already in there. It's already painful. It's already being dealt with by being repressed or supressed, and therefore it's harming you. It's creating harm and the way it's doing it, is because It's affecting how you are processing information today.

Mm.

Does that make sense?

Yeah.

Therefore, the way you are processing information is less than optimal. There has not been a successful resolution of these negative feelings. Negative feelings always point to a need, and then you think, 'Okay, this is grief about loss or something. What do I need? There is nothing I can do to change it, so it's time to let go of it.' But you can't let go of it if it is being repressed or supressed.

Mm.

But the very nature is to deny it: denial, denial. And that keeps you and quite often people will, they will go through this process 'Oh, I feel pain. My denial has been shattered,' and that's what happens as we are going through this, your denial is shattered. The anger got released but there is nothing you can do with the anger so it stays inside and that's what is giving you that sensation of heaviness, of sadness: it's unre-solved grief.

Yeah I just feel, I feel so exhausted.

It is exhausting and this is why I will always start the sessions by saying what would you like to talk about today? And you might say, 'Well, actually I would like to talk about politics today because that way I can put it out there and I don't have to deal with all that shit in the AAI.'

But I am glad, Charley, that I have said what I wanted to talk about today. I am still glad I have made that decision even though I am feeling really shat-tered. I'm I feel pleased that I've bitten the bullet.

Yeah.

Yeah it feels hard and I feel—like today I feel like I can't really do any more. I feel I've reached saturation point with it, but I know that, next time, all being well, I will be ready to start again, and the way that you are doing it, I do feel... that it, it feels very, erm, patient.

Mm.

The way you are handling, the way you are handling the transcript, it feels patient. It feels there is a lot to do, but patiently. And I feel like I will be able to deal with it and I am dealing with it and that's all fine, but I just feel … incredibly tired, and I suppose it's dealing with this and all the other shit in my life that tires me out, you know? All the problems with my children and my ex-husband etc, etc, so I suppose I'm just worn out.

Yeah, and that's where, that's why this is so important is because all this unresolved stuff in the past makes dealing with these current problems and challenges harder.

Mm.

And you might say, 'Well, why? How is this making it easier? It's just piling more stuff on.'

I don't see it like that

Okay, good. That's what I wanted to check out.

I don't see it like that. I see it as, erm, as—completing the jigsaw. The pieces that are missing. The pieces I can't remember and the things I want to go back and maybe have some answers for, so I see it as a positive thing. You learn something different about yourself and it's a revelation, and that's fascinating.

A Year Later

Here she is a year later. We have been working through the section about her father:

Is there anything that you want to add or modify, thinking where you are with it today?

There is nothing more that I want to add, apart from, I would say that certainly over the last couple of months, a lot of things are making a lot more sense to me and slotted into place, if that makes sense?

Yeah. Can you give me an example of that?

I think, erm an example is working through this process with the questions, hearing what I said, and hearing what I am saying again today is actually very helpful. And when I am saying what I am saying today, I am sort of, things are whirling around and erm, it's almost as if some things do feel resolved *as* I am saying them if that makes sense?

Yeah, absolutely. I'm glad.

Yeah. I think that's why I am so keen to, to keep going with the transcript, because it is concentrating on me, and I am understanding how so many things fit in to my whole life that make, um—that make sense. There are, obviously, there are big chunks that I can't remember and I am actually wondering does it actually matter that I can't remember any more? Does that matter? I don't really think it does erm, not really.

Well, you've asked err a very important question. Erm does it or doesn't it? Let's reflect on that a bit. Honestly, I don't know the answer to that question because I, I think that it's err—it's a very personal kind of proposition, so rather than does it matter in an abstract sense, the important question is, does it matter to you? Does it make a difference in your life?

Sometimes it does matter to me Charley, but to answer the question, does it make a difference in my life? No it doesn't. It doesn't because my life is now. My life is about moving forward and I'm very keen, in a way, to work through this transcript as thoroughly as I can, but as swiftly as I can in another way, because, to me, this is so, such a positive thing to do because my moving on at a—a steady pace, it feels like I am moving on and putting the past in a place where it needs to be so that I can concentrate on the future. So for me, the whole thing is incredible. Erm, it's actually very healing. The whole thing is very healing just to talk about it, and to talk about it in the context is far more beneficial to go through this interview, than just to willy nilly turn up to a counselling session and talk about any old crap. This, to me, feels like there is a lot more purpose behind it and structure rather than airy fairy, no offence, counselling shit. So I am genuinely relishing moving through the questions and thinking about how they are making me feel.

There are lots that I could say about these two excerpts. However, the point is not to focus on the content but rather the process, which is what we do in coding the AAI, as well. While what is said, the history, is important, what is more important is how it is said. It is also that what we find early on are clues, and while we may speculate as to the meaning, we don't have enough information yet to be very certain about anything. As we go further into the transcript and learn more about how the client is processing information, we can deduce further meaning, as the next excerpt demonstrates.

REHAN'S LOVER

This is an excerpt from Rehan's AAI in which we can see the A+ tendency to rationalize, idealize, and give a positive spin to the emotional deprivation that they suffered as children. This excerpt illustrates how the lack of comfort, physical and emotional abuse, shifting roles and responsibilities set Rehan up for serious problems in adulthood.

Unlike the previous example, this is not a recording of a session where we go through the AAI together. It is based on my recollection of my interpretations as I went through it with Rehan. The enigmatic response regarding what Rehan did when he was emotionally upset Rehan clarified when queried for this book, as you will read. Likewise, Rehan confirmed the information about his father's physical abuse and kicking him while he lay on the doorstep.

Also, I often speak from a place of certainty. But this needs to be understood as, 'I am certain that, right now, this is my hypothesis.' I am never *certain* that my hypothesis is correct. I stress to clients that if they disagree, to please say so.

Rehan was 39 years old when he first came to see me. He was married, with children, and had a lover on the side. This conflicted with his religious family background. He had become accustomed to not getting his needs met. Religion can be a convenient justification for the harsh parenting style that Rehan experienced. This lack of getting needs met had contributed to him getting into his marriage. They were both in the same religious sect and so they were marrying, not because they were attracted to one another physically, emotionally, and spiritually, but because it was the 'right' thing to do. There had been no sexual intercourse and no 'heavy petting' prior to marriage. He had not anticipated that the marriage would never be physically or emotionally satisfying to him. This pattern suggests an A8, externally assembled self, strategy. Like many using an A5–6 strategy, which are lower numbered but are typically included in the higher numbered strategies, he turned to sex outside the marriage as a way to make up for unmet emotional needs. He was also self-harming (cutting) and often thought of suicide.

This excerpt reflects the lack of comfort in childhood. Remember that these events are not *causation*, although they will contribute to keeping the causation ball rolling that had begun in infancy and early childhood.

> **What about when you were hurt physically, what would you do?**
> Erm? ... (14) [the dots and the number denote a 14 second pause] (sighs) [the sigh is indicative of sadness] I remember falling off, off ... [the cut-off and repetition of 'off' are dysfluencies that indicate a repressed emotion associated with this event] a skateboard once and really kind of ['kind of' softens the impact by minimizing and making it equivocal] going through my trousers and down to my knee. And the thing that I remember is that I damaged the trousers and that was another pair of tracksuit trousers that I had damaged, rather than anything else—erm, yeah.

Rehan is focused on the damage to a pair of trousers rather than to himself. This reflects learned behaviour: to put things and not displeasing his parents above his own needs and feelings. Rehan can state that as a fact, yet the emotional conclusion—or the metacognition about what he is saying—is missing.

> **You remember what happened afterwards?**
> No, no—erm no—

Lack of memory is a common feature of the A strategy. By not 'remembering,' the negative emotions are avoided. Emotions are the primary memory access route, which is why C's are able to give so many detailed memories.

> **Okay**
> I don't remember any specific—I don't remember feeling particularly like—I don't know, don't know.

Again, there is a failure of memory. The details and the overall emotional tone are missing. Notice that the cut-offs after 'specific' and 'like' prevent him even articulating the word 'feelings.'

> **So, if you were upset emotionally what would you do?**
> Erm, I would talk to my mum.
> **Mm-hmm**
> rather than my Dad—erm,
> **What would—what would Mom do?**
> Erm? Can't … listen, give advice erm. (4)

The 'erm' appears to be stalling as he thinks how to answer. It is not clear what 'can't' refers to. Perhaps he was going to say, 'can't remember,' but he doesn't say that. He cuts off whatever he was going to say and instead, if we ignore the pause we get: 'Can't listen, [or] give advice, erm.' Alternatively, it could have been, 'Can't listen because she is too busy giving advice.' We don't know. Rehan perhaps 'knows,' at an unconscious mind level, but he can't bring himself to say it and make it conscious.

(Note: As I am still working with Rehan, and we are some years down the road, I asked him what he meant by this answer. He explained it this way:

I would go in on myself, get very anxious and worried, believe that whatever happened was my fault, that I was to blame. If it got to be unbearable I would go to my mom. Mom would try and offer some reassurance, but in a way that meant I would pick up her anxiety about whatever I was sharing. She would listen and offer advice but she wouldn't reassure me. She might offer to pray about it, but in a way that made me feel that it was my fault.

The first thing I notice about this answer is that it is a coherent narrative of his experience. It is balanced in that he articulates his role in the interaction and both the good and bad aspects of mom's attempts at reassurance, acknowledging her good intentions but also noticing that they paved the road to his own internal hell, of believing that, whatever it was, it was his fault. This inherent sense of fault becomes shame, which led to his self-harm and suicidal ideation. I also notice that it is a more nuanced and richer explanation than the either/or dichotomy that I had hypothesized.)

Rehan was very distressed being asked about what he did when he needed comfort, as evidenced by the next question:

> **Okay.**
> Yeah
> **Okay. If you needed comfort what would you do?**
> If I—sorry if I was?

Here Rehan asks me to repeat the question. It is simple, not hard to understand. Is it because he is so distraught from the previous question that he cannot take in this question? Rehan's emotions seem to be so turbulent that they have interfered with not only his ability to answer the previous question but his ability to hear the present question. I repeat:

> **If you needed comfort?**
> If I was?—yeah, they would have given me a hug.

The unconscious mind has the information, but the filtering process won't let it come through. But because there is pressure for the information to come through—the unconscious mind would like nothing better than to be able to resolve these dilemmas and get rid of negative emotions from the past if it just knew how—the filtering creates resistance and thus turbulence in the flow of information: dysfluency of discourse and information processing of both thoughts and feelings.

This is where another aspect of Grice's Cooperative Principle comes into play. As listeners, we automatically correct for the manner of the discourse. If we use our top-down knowledge base, we miss the true meaning: 'My mother couldn't listen to me when I was emotionally upset and even if she had of done she would not have been able to help me deal with it.' By using the DMM discourse analysis, which dovetails nicely with NLP in terms of looking for hidden unconscious meanings, we can make sense of nonsense, we can form a hypothesis of what the client's experience was and help them to elicit the missing pieces.

Rehan's top-down model meant that this was an unacceptable thing to say about his mother, whom he ought, as a 'good boy,' to love and say nothing bad about. This is a rather superficial filter—beliefs filter our information, some is excluded, other is distorted, coloured, spun, what have you—and it conflicts with the information he actually has. That filter, or belief, will be rather easy to challenge using Rational Emotive Behaviour Therapy (REBT). It may take a while because that belief was probably instilled very young, pre-school.

Oh Shit! I'm Gonna Die Now!

There is almost certainly a much more fundamental filter, buried very deeply, and connecting directly to our life support system. That belief is that if Mom and Dad desert me, I will die, and if I am not a good boy, then they will desert me, and being critical of my mom's parenting will make me not a good boy. But the fundamental fear is, 'Oh shit, I'm gonna die now.' It could be because of the wolf in the closet that's going to jump out and eat you at any moment, or because if your parents don't feed you, you will starve to death, or if they throw you out on a cold night you could freeze to death, that you would die. But your primitive brain, your life support system, is pre-programmed with one central belief towards which all of your energy can be directed, and it is this: without their care I will die. And that's the truth.

But this is only true in the early years. As children get older, they become more capable of taking care of themselves, whatever the parenting they received. There are many stories of children existing, living, however they can. *Oliver!*[2] Is a romanticized version of this phenomenon.

Also, in our culture, if a child was to be abandoned by parents, then it is likely that someone would step in to care for them. It is easy for us to be oblivious to the mortal fear that a child feels when left alone or threatened with abandonment.

So, even though children learn, at a cognitive level, how to make their way in the world even with missing or impaired caregivers, they nevertheless remain bound, as older children and adults, by the emotional bonds created by that early programming. Let's consider an elephant, fully grown, that is standing next to a stake in the ground with a puny chain from the stake around a ring, or cuff, on one of the elephant's front legs. Now, as we look, we notice something a bit strange: the stake and chain seem inadequate to the task of restraining this full-grown elephant. Why doesn't the elephant simply yank it out and run away?

Learned Helplessness

Martin Seligman[3] coined the term 'learned helplessness.' Seligman put puppies in cages. He then administered a mild electrical shock to the bottom of the cages. The dogs were not injured, we are assured—except psychologically and emotionally, as we shall see—but the shock was sufficient to motivate them to want to get away, because it hurt and it was, well, a shock. But they couldn't get away. They could only sit and whimper at the pain. I suppose they may have peed, too, knowing puppies. He did this every day for a few weeks and then left the dogs to grow into adults.

He then brought them back for more shocking treatment. But there was a catch: the cages the dogs were in had no tops on them. They were the same cages that they had been put in as puppies, only then, the puppies were too small to be able to jump out of the cages. But now, they were grown and could have easily jumped out of the cages. But they didn't. Seligman's theory, which he dubbed 'learned helplessness,' was that the dogs, as puppies, had learned to be helpless in this scenario, and so the emotional programming of this learning left them emotionally unable to do what they were perfectly well capable of doing physically.

In the same way, the mahouts of India train the baby elephant by chaining them by the leg to the stake when they are small, and they 'learn' that they can't get free of the chain and stake, and so, after a while, they stop trying. That's why they stand placidly by a stake and chain manifestly too small to hold them physically: they are bound by stronger bonds emotionally.

Even though consciously Rehan no longer believes that he will die if abandoned by his caregivers, the part of his unconscious mind that is responsible for his survival, the life support system, moderated via the limbic, or learning, system, was still acting as if it was true. Unfortunately, the behaviour that he had learned as a child as a way to cope and preserve his life was threatening his life as an adult. The intolerable conflict between the evidence of his senses and his cognition with his emotional programming was threatening to kill him now.

In addition to the self-harm of cutting, he also had frequent bouts of depression accompanied by suicidal thoughts. These thoughts were comforting because the thought of ending the pain—and existence—was comforting to him in the perverse way that removal of pain is a comfort even if it means ending one's life.

Back to Rehan's discourse: for his benefit I repeated the question:

If you needed comfort?
If I was—yeah, they would have given me a hug.

I talked Rehan through my analysis of his discourse. I thought that he was so emotionally embroiled in the previous question that he did not hear, nor could he respond to, the next question until it had been repeated. His answer to the question was in a hypothetical 'if/then' construction. So, to take his last sentence and reinterpret it: 'If I was [in need of comfort] (notice here that he could not even say those words, he substitutes "yeah", a nonsense word) [then] they *would have given* [italics added] me a hug.' 'But of course I never needed a hug, or comfort,' he might have added. A's learn to deny their need for comfort. So what apparently was a positive reply comes across as Rehan's need to put a positive gloss on his childhood. We call this 'false positive affect.' Rehan confessed he could not remember actually getting a hug. His answer was based on what he thought a parent 'should' do.

I can only form a hypothesis and test it, and I can only know if I am right if the client can confirm it. There is always the danger that a client might agree because they want to please me, the therapist. I do what I can to guard against this. First off, I encourage clients to disagree with my interpretation. I explain to them that no matter what I think or whether I am right or wrong, the information is only useful to them if they can use it. It needs to resonate with what they innately know to be true or have some explanatory value that is useful to them in understanding their behaviour and the behaviour of others. More important, it needs to be useful in helping them to change for the better.

My interpretations, insights, or analyses are offered as advisory opinions only. However, I have found that these interpretations often give the client permission to feel, think, and understand things that they have been denying or avoiding, even repressing, for a long time. If my interpretation is wrong, then the feedback from the client as to why it is wrong gives new information that we add into the process. This is the recursive nature of ACT. In answer to the question regarding his childhood relationship with his mother, he says:

> R: Okay. Erm? I—my mum was at home when we were younger, erm and then as she was due—she started to go back into work. That's when she became ill so she was around a lot. I remember on—on the one hand I think my mum being quite erm, affectionate with us but there—there was always a sense of err, even from very young, us needing to—or needing to be a certain way, behave in a certain way erm, to—in order to kind of get approval to be seen to be erm, be seen to be—erm, yeah. It's kind of the public face of the family is quite important so it's important that I was successful at school. It was important that I behaved in a certain way in public. That, that kind of thing was—was very significant to my mum. Erm—I—I—my relationship with my mum was much closer or is much closer with my relationship with my Dad. Erm there was a lot of arguments and conflicts between my mum and my Dad, my Dad and my sister, particularly growing up, erm, and I would often take the role of peacemaker and try and negotiate between different people in order to try and bring some sort of peace and harmony, erm, and that certainly is, is a memory that I have got going way back erm—yeah. (sigh) Erm … (3) and my mum—I think my mum has increasingly tried to express erm, her—her being pleased with whatever, we, we have chosen to do being you know later days, later times, but, erm, I think there is that kind of nagging sense of that was still very much, that was what was important and my role of being able to kind of bring about kind of resolution of conflict within the family erm … My relationship with my dad wasn't particularly close, my dad struggled to really show much interest in things that he didn't have an interest in himself. Erm, he's—he is quite a kind of Aspergersy—quite autistically type character in some ways but yeah. And just—you had to kind of find a way of being interested in something that he was interested in in order for him to, erm want to sort of engage if you like **mm** erm so.

The most noticeable feature is the dysfluency. You may also notice that he cannot talk about Mom without talking about his Dad *and* his sister. He finds some complimentary things to say about his relationship with Mom, but only in comparison to his very withdrawn and angry father. This is an indicator from within the interview structure of triangulation. In this scenario Rehan describes himself as being the peacemaker. This is role reversal: Rehan is playing the role of peacemaker in the family in the place of his parents, who seem to be squabbling like children in his recounting of it.

Another indicator of Rehan's A strategy, at least in relation to me in this interview, was this exchange about the words used to describe the childhood relationship with Dad:

> **Has [another one] come to mind?**
> Erm yes, yeah—erm anger, angry,
> **Oh, okay. Oh, we skipped anger, we skipped anger [at this point I realized that I had made an error in the interviewing process: I had overlooked the word, anger.]**
> I wondered if I had said.
> **No, it's my fault. Sorry. [obviously it was my mistake as I had written the word down but had overlooked it, duh!]**
> No, no I—erm—yeah, yeah it.

Notice how Rehan responds to a mistake having been made: he immediately and instinctively tries to take the blame for the mistake onto himself! Even protesting when I point out that it was *my* error, not his.

Going on, he describes dad's anger:

> He would, he would go from very calm to very, very angry very quickly erm—so I remember him, lots of occasions where he would swear at my mum, swear at me, swear at my sister. **mm** I remember him throwing things through a window once erm—I remember being kicked on, you know, on occasion on the doorstep. Erm he would get very, very angry very quickly erm, **mm** and then it would—it would then take a long time for things to kind of calm back down again afterwards. Erm, but, yeah—that would— that, that would often punctuate the mealtimes were often kind of quite fiery occasions erm, but yeah.

In this paragraph, notice repetition of 'very, very angry very quickly,' and within the phrase the repetition of 'very.' It might to tempting to interpret this as a C type repetition: evocative language. However, this may instead be trauma talking. Notice the last sentence is not grammatically correct. And pay particular attention to, 'I remember being kicked on, you know, on occasion, on the doorstep.' Notice the blandness implied by the phrase, 'on occasion.'

When we examine this sentence carefully, we can notice the extreme repression of feelings. When Rehan says, 'I remember being kicked on … the doorstep,' it becomes nonsensical. That is to say, Rehan doesn't have a body part called 'the doorstep.' He has shins that he could have been kicked on or a butt that he could have been kicked on, but not a doorstep.

When we use Grice's Maxim of quality and manner to automatically correct, it goes by unnoticed. But when we consider it mindfully, we understand 'being kicked on the doorstep,' as referring to a physical location. So now we realize that some information is missing. We then ask ourselves, if Rehan was on the doorstep, what was he doing there? Was he in the way and dad wanted to go through the door and that is why dad kicked Rehan? How bad was the kick? Was it a gentle nudge to get him to move? A 'C' strategist might describe that as being 'kicked.' And what is the significance of stating the physical location of the doorstep without explanation? We might expect, 'I was standing on the doorstep and my dad wanted to get by and got angry, so he kicked me.'

Fortunately, using the AAI as I do, and going through it with the client, I can ask him to explain, which I did. What emerged is that Rehan wasn't *standing* on the doorstep, he was *lying* on the doorstep. When asked how he came to be lying on the doorstep—not a particularly appealing place to be lounging about—Rehan explained that his father had placed him there. In other words, dad had knocked him down onto the front doorstep and started kicking him while he was down! Literally.

That's quite a different story from the matter-of-fact manner in which Rehan told the story in the AAI. But the clues are there.

At another point Rehan is explaining why he felt closer to Mom than to Dad:

Erm? I think I—(sighs) there was some warmth from my mom. I think I probably understood a bit more about how to get—praise and affection and attention from my mum. Erm—I think my—in some way my personality was more attuned to my mum's than my dad's—my sister was very much like my dad, people would always say, you know, 'You are just like your mum and my sister was just like my dad,'—erm—so I suppose there was more of that kind of similarity there.

Rehan sees it as his responsibility to be able to elicit caregiving from his parents. Mom was better at caregiving because he, Rehan, knew better how to make it happen. Dad was inadequate because Rehan didn't know how to elicit caregiving from his father. This is self-responsibility, which often accompanies role reversal.

He then compares personalities, which is exoneration for dad. However, his statement comparing personalities does not make sense either. Here it is: 'You are just like your mum and my sister was just like my dad.' Now imagine that you are the speaker saying that to Rehan. It would be correct if we were comparing families: you, Rehan, being like your mom, and my sister, Sandra, being just like my dad. Again, Grice's Maxims, while they help us to understand one another, will have misled us unless we are mindful of them. In this case, you might say to me, 'Don't be silly, Charley. It is obvious that Rehan is talking about *his* sister and *his* dad.' Yes, using Grice's Maxims, it does become obvious. But analysing it as we have done, we notice something extremely important: the perspective of the speaker changes without Rehan being aware of it. He shifts from the third-person speaker who is saying to Rehan, '*You* are just like your mom,' to himself, '*my* sister was just like my dad.' This is not hugely incoherent, hence we might have missed it. But an unaware shifting of perspective is extremely important. Again, it indicates errors of information processing. The 'you' is distanced: someone else is saying that about Rehan, our speaker. But 'my' is personal. We might suspect that Rehan can feel closer to his sister than he can to himself. This could be an example of Rehan being dismissing of himself and preoccupied with the needs of others.

Mom's inadequate caregiving Rehan 'explains' to himself as being due to his own inadequacies in eliciting caregiving and the personality differences. This reinforces his sense of worthlessness of deserving anything better. This constitutes shame. Hence, his negative feelings have been turned inwards upon himself in a variety of ways, manifested most extremely by his self-harm and his suicidal ideation, and in other ways less obvious.

In this case, there was something in the process that allowed Rehan to spontaneously acknowledge the loathing that he felt for his parents. In one of our sessions, he described seeing them in person as 'ripping the scab off a wound that never healed.' I inquired into why that wound had never healed. I allowed that he kept wounding himself, literally, as a way to displace the pain and anger that he felt towards his parents. He acknowledged that he would prefer never to see them again.

We will return to Rehan and his lover later on. As Rehan has made progress in the core beliefs, and as he has dealt with the guilt and grief equation, he has come to a place of acceptance that his parents did the best they could do, and so he is at peace with them. Now he only has his wife and his girlfriend to deal with!

NOTES

1. Crittenden, P. M., & Landini, A. (2011). *Assessing adult attachment: A dynamic-maturational approach to discourse analysis.* WW Norton & Company.
2. https://en.wikipedia.org/wiki/Oliver!_(film).
3. https://en.wikipedia.org/wiki/Learned_helplessness.

CHAPTER 5

Rational Emotive Behaviour Therapy

Words are more than mere symbols.
They are the tools we use to grasp and grapple with reality.
—Anonymous *(I wish I knew to whom to credit this quote. I heard it*
on a program about dyslexia. I have since tried to find it to give proper
credit. I have not been able to do so. If anyone knows,
please let me know.)

The beginning of wisdom is to call things by their right name.
—Confucius

Rational Emotive Behaviour Therapy (REBT) depends on calling things by their right names. It is the original and in my opinion the best form of Cognitive Behavioural Therapy (CBT).[1] REBT is, unfortunately, often misunderstood and often misapplied even by clinicians. I have had many clients who had previously experienced CBT and found it lacking. That is because, as a stand-alone therapy, it is unlikely to be successful. It has certain specific uses for which it is appropriate and others where it is misplaced. REBT is a *tool*. As such, it enables us to do a job, a task. But it is not likely to be the only tool we need. If you want to build a house, you will need more than a hammer.

You will also notice in later examples plenty of places where REBT *could* be used, but the opportunity is ignored. That is because, in my judgement,

C. Shults, *Attachment Centred Therapy*, Palgrave Texts in Counselling and Psychotherapy, https://doi.org/10.1007/978-3-031-60851-3_5

that was not the point. I don't point these out, but if you look for them you will find them. There will be other places where it is important, in my judgement, and so I persist in trying to get the client to look at what their belief is, what they are telling themselves about what is going on. And when I say judgement, that is not meant only in the sense of it being a judgement by the therapist about which is the most useful to pursue.

I place it here because it is a systematic way to challenge irrational beliefs that lead to mal-adaptive behaviours. These irrational beliefs are a type of error in information processing, and so are an integral part of attachment strategies. We have already seen the mal-adaptive core belief, 'I am a bad, unworthy person.' This was inherent in the previous example of Rehan. This is at the root of many people's difficulties and is directly related to unmet attachment needs. We could jump immediately to the affirmation, 'I am a good, worthwhile person.' If your client is ready to go there, then by all means do. However, in terms of Grice's Maxims, we might be violating quality, as there is not yet a firm evidentiary basis for the truth of that affirmation. Going through the REBT process is teaching the client how to use the process. We will see that in action later in this chapter.

The ABCs of Emotions

REBT uses the mnemonic, ABCDE, to remember the steps. The A is the activating event that sets the process in motion. This is something that happens to us, to someone we love, to someone we hate, or any event in which we have an interest. B is the belief that our mind applies to this situation. Sometimes it isn't obvious what the belief is, and we have to do a bit of digging. Many of our beliefs are buried so deeply that we take them for granted, not realizing that they were what we were taught in childhood, before conscious memory formation. C is the consequence: our emotional and behavioural response. We can have very different responses to the same situation depending on our belief about the event. This consequence can be a feeling state (fear), a behaviour (running away), or both, and a combination of the two as when a behavioural impulse is described as a feeling state: 'I feel like running away.'

The trouble with a statement that uses a behavioural description to describe a feeling state is that it does not always elicit caregiving. For example, Racine, after she had broken up with John, felt uncomfortable with being in his presence because he was being very punitive towards her. This discomfort was great, and she expressed it to her mother as 'I want to leave that college. I don't want to go there anymore.' What she was really trying to express was her feeling of discomfort at having to be around John. Her goal in expressing this to her mother was to elicit comfort. Her mother, being a good performance-oriented A+, was alarmed by her daughter's apparent disregard for the importance of education above all else. This alarm then prevented mother from giving daughter the support and comfort that she needed. She reacted negatively because she heard her daughter literally, as A's often do when C's express their negative emotion in behavioural terms.

In this technique, once the B, the belief, is identified, we then apply three questions to this belief.

THREE QUESTIONS

1. Does this belief help me to deal with the situation?
2. Is this belief based on known facts and reality?
3. Is this belief logical?

These are straightforward questions, but clients may have a bit of difficulty with them. In order to be a 'rational' belief it has to pass all three with a 'yes.'

The first question is pragmatic. Does it help or doesn't it? Let's take a commonly held belief: 'I can't bring up difficult topics with my partner because it will just cause a row.' The belief is helpful, one might argue, because it avoids an argument. This belief is common with the A strategy. Short term, it does help for the stated reason: it avoids an argument, hence the label 'avoidant.' But long term it is far from helpful. The A's feelings are not dealt with effectively, needs are not met, resentments accumulate, frustrations build, and the likelihood of a blow up later on grows.

Next is, 'Is the belief based on known facts and reality?' The client might say, 'Yes, it is based on the facts and reality that I know. That's what it was like growing up, and that is what I experience with my partner. Bringing up difficult topics just causes trouble.' These instances acknowledge that this is consistent with the client's reality. But then look at the bigger picture to see that, in general, it is not consistent with known facts and reality. I meet the maxim of quality by referencing the research into what makes couples happy.[2]

The third question, is it logical, tends to answer itself. If a belief doesn't help to deal with the situation and isn't based on known facts and reality, then it isn't logical to continue with that belief. While it is not likely, I have occasionally encountered a belief that could pass the first two but fail on the third test.

When the belief has failed on one or more of these questions, then we go on to the D part: dispute the irrational belief.

The disputation for the first question might be, 'Yes, not discussing difficult topics helps me in the short term, but long term it makes things worse because problems aren't addressed. It will be better for me to learn how to express my thoughts and feelings in an appropriate manner. In the long run this will make us both happier.'

The disputation for the second question might be, 'Yes, that was my experience growing up, and I have replicated it in my current attachment relationship. But I know from the results that I've got and the things that I am learning that it is not a good idea. The reality is that it is better to learn how to work things out instead of avoiding them.'

The disputation for the third question might be, 'It is crazy for me to continue to hang on to that belief since it is illogical. Adopting a more logical belief will help me to get my needs met in the long run and help us both to be happier.'

I have compiled these five steps of REBT: Activating Event, Belief, Consequence, Disputing the Irrational Belief, and Effective Emotional Response; into a single worksheet that I share with you as Appendix A.

In order for REBT to be most effective, we need to practise it until it becomes reflexive. You can't learn to roll a kayak in the middle of a rapid, and you can't learn to use REBT in the middle of an argument. We need to practise it so often that when we have an emotion, in terms of feelings or behaviour, we *automatically* look for the accompanying belief, challenge that belief with the three questions, and if it fails for any reason, immediately begin to search for a better, *rational* belief that passes muster on our three questions.

Since C's distort cognitive information, to include eliminating it completely other than to reinforce emotions, REBT needs to be a significant factor in working with the C strategy. A few caveats are in order here. First, people tend to feel more comfortable going with their strengths. This is due to the economy of effort needed to restate what we already believe. It takes much more effort to change a belief than it does to reiterate it. It is also easier and more comfortable to hang on to old beliefs and behaviours. Thus, the very thing that the client needs to change, their reliance on how they *feel* about something, militates against the very thing they need to do to correct it. That doesn't mean that one needn't try. What it means is that one must make an emotional argument in favour of using a cognitive approach. The saying that I came up with for C's is:

Emotionally, it feels good to be more logical.

REBT is also useful for A's. Even though A's already overly rely on their cognition in making decisions, many of their beliefs are distorted, and the higher the numbers, the more the distortion. These primarily fit into the category of their own needs and feelings not being important enough to assert. This is typically associated with and emanates from a core belief of unworthiness, hence the 'I am a bad, unworthy person' core belief filters their perceptions and motivates their behaviour. While C's use distorted information processing in the form of irrational beliefs to justify their position, so do A's. They just use them in different ways and for different purposes. The saying for A's is:

Logically, it makes sense to be more emotional.

Why does it make sense? Because emotions *motivate*. Without motivation, little is accomplished.

REBT does not ask where the belief came from, and why is it held onto as if life itself depended on it. That is where ACT comes in. When we follow this trail, it leads us straight back to those early attachment experiences and our model of the world that we inherited from our caregivers.

Two Tips to Training Thinking

There are two tips that you can use to facilitate thinking about and learning the REBT system. They are 'shoulds' and 'hot links.' As these two ideas have to do with specific words and patterns, they are easily learned and practised. I recommend learning these well and attaching a warning bell, bright flashing lights, and maybe a rumble strip to each of these so that you are alerted that any time you use them, trouble is likely to lie ahead.

'Shoulds'

One of the things we were taught to look out for in early recovery from addiction is 'numerous shoulds.' That is, people who were suffering from an addictive disorder often had numerous 'shoulds' that they put on themselves. They 'shouldn't' (a negation is still a 'should') drink so much. They should be a better person. They should visit their mother more often. They shouldn't look at so much porn. They should go to church more often. They shouldn't spend their pay check on crack cocaine.

Unfortunately, those 'shoulds' never changed the person's behaviour. In fact, it seemed to make it worse. Why? Because 'shoulds' are shaming. And the more shame we feel, the more motivated to do the addictive or otherwise dysfunctional behaviour to relieve our shame.

Let's examine the proper use of the word 'should.' When we use it as a conditional, 'It should rain tomorrow [if the weather report is correct].' The words in brackets are not spoken but are understood. 'You should ace that test tomorrow,' can be understood in two ways. In one sense it could mean: 'You are under an obligation to do well on the test tomorrow and if you don't you "should" be ashamed because you are letting down all the people who are counting on you.' Or it could mean, 'Judging by your past performance on this type of exam, and considering the amount of preparation you have put in, you should [will probably] do very well on the exam tomorrow.' The latter sense is justified, again, as a contingency or prediction. The former sense is shaming.

So, for example, a statement such as 'You should be more like your sister' is inherently and intentionally shaming. Not good.

'You mean you don't know how to do that and you're 8 years old? Why you should be able to do that by now.' One can argue that in one sense it is not shaming. In that case, make your intention clear by saying, 'You mean you don't know how to do that? Well, I need to teach you how, in that case.' The other sense is clearly and completely shaming: the message is, 'You are somehow inferior for not knowing how to do that task, and I am completely exonerated of any responsibility for teaching you.'

'Should' statements of this latter variety will virtually never be rational. I recommend you test it as much as you like in order to be convinced.

'Should' and 'must' are synonymous in REBT. 'Must' was one of Ellis' favourite words to avoid. The use of the word was associated with what Ellis dubbed 'mustubatory behaviour.' He used the examples of 'I must,' 'You must,' or 'The world must' be or behave in a certain way in order for me to be satisfied, happy, content, vindicated, replicated, etcetera-ted. These are conditions and expectations placed on people and events that lead to unpleasant emotions through what Ellis called 'hot links' that we will look at in the next section. What Ellis advocated instead was USA (unconditional self-acceptance) and UOA (unconditional other acceptance).

You may have already realized that this system has something in common with yogic philosophy and Buddhism, in that it is 'attachment' to things, beliefs, people, that causes suffering (negative emotions). You can also relate it to letting go of expectations that we will examine in the section on meditation.

The same with the word 'ought.' It can be used synonymously with 'should.' So we ought to get rid of it and we should never use it. We must avoid all three words at all cost: should, must, and ought.

Remember:

Don't 'should' on yourself today!

What to Do Instead?
Instead of 'shoulding' on yourself or others (or 'musturbating' or 'oughting'), try substituting need, will, desire, or ability:

> Instead of, 'You should be able to do that,' try: 'It's time for you to learn … I need to show you how.'
> Instead of, 'It must be done this way,' try, 'My preference is this way, but you can do it however you like to get the job done.'
> Instead of, 'You ought to apply for that job (or study now, or whatever),' try, 'There's a job opening if you are interested,' or, 'It's up to you how much you want to study for the exam. However, if you want to do your best, you need to prepare.'

I'm sure there are many ways to communicate that don't require 'should,' 'ought,' of 'must.' You can find them, I'm sure.

Of course, there are also legitimate uses for these words. 'I must get this job done if I am to be impeccable with my word.' 'I really should check that out instead of making assumptions.' 'I ought to prepare for my test.'

Hot Links

Hot links are the words that we automatically use to put ourselves and others down. These provide the link between the event (A=activating event) and the consequence (C = behaviours and feelings) by characterizing the belief (B=belief). Those characterizations (or what we tell ourselves) come in five flavours: condemnation and damnation, I-can't-stand-it-itis, awfulizing, self-downing, and always/never.

I have a little statement that encapsulates the five: 'Goddammit, I can't stand it! It's so awful! I'll never be good enough! I'll always screw it up!'

Let's take them in order.

Condemnation and Damnation

This is inherently shaming. It can be very tempting because it can feel so good to release those pent-up emotions in a negative way that puts all the blame elsewhere. And because it feels so good, we can become addicted to it, habituated, so that it just comes out automatically.

I-Can't-Stand-It-Itis

As the name implies, I can't stand it: when things don't go my way; when people won't do what I want them to; when the government tells me I have to stay at home or wear a mask; when my team loses; when immigrants move in next door; when my kid slams the door; when my baby don't want me no more.

The I-can't-stand-it automatic response discounts our ability to cope and denies the possibility of accepting the reality of the way things are.

The thing is, there are plenty of things that we ought (as in, owe it to ourselves and others) to find unacceptable, and therefore, we need to be able to marshal our angry energy towards changing. But I-can't-stand-it denies our ability to change it.

'I don't like it, I don't think it's right, or just, or fair, and therefore I intend to do what I can change it,' is a much better attitude to take.

Awfulizing

'Ain't it awful?'

Well, probably not. It may be inconvenient, undesirable, or unhelpful, but it's not necessarily awful. The surest test of whether or not a word is appropriate is to use the three questions to determine rationality: does it help to deal with the situation; is it based on known facts and reality; is it logical? Some things are very bad and can appropriately be described as awful.

On the other hand, your favourite actor not winning an Oscar is not 'awful.'

Self-downing

Self-downing is never a good idea. That's why, every time I do it, I tell myself how stupid I am! No, just kidding.

There is another joke of that nature in the REBT workbook. The task is to divide statements into the A, B, Cs. One of the statements is, 'I feel really put down; I can't understand this therapy. This proves how inadequate I am.' The joke is that a process that is meant to be helpful can actually be twisted around into something that makes the problem worse by using one of the hot links. You may find that your clients have a tendency to do this. Gentle encouragement is in order.

Always/Never
And finally, last but by no means least, my personal all-time favourite, the one I always use, that never fails: always/nevering. These are the two words that you always want to avoid and you never want to use. Unless, of course, they are totally appropriate, which, in the normal course of conversation, they almost never are.

When always/never statements are used in marital arguments, it usually is inaccurate. So, when one partner says to another, 'You always,' or 'You never,' it is likely to be inaccurate to one degree or another. Stating the case in extremes may have dramatic appeal, but eventually the other partner is going to become resentful of having their efforts discounted.

THE ZIGZAG

Old beliefs die hard. They may persist no matter how rational your new beliefs are. This is where the zigzag technique comes in. This gives you a method to reinforce your new belief and make it stronger.

Start with the new belief and write it at the top left corner of the page. Then you give a rating of conviction: that is the degree to which you can actually *wholeheartedly* believe this new belief, on a scale of 0–100. Then go to the right-hand side of the page, a little lower down and write down your objections, or attack, to this new belief.

Next, go to the left-hand side of the page and make a new box below the first one where you now write your response to the attack. Use the response to answer each point made in the attack. Once this has been done, check to see if there are other objections, or attacks, that the inner critic wants to make. If so, write them down in another box on the right-hand side. Then repeat the process of responding to each new attack. Do this as many times as necessary. Be sure to end on the left-hand side of the page with a positive response. Then end the exercise by giving yourself a new rating of the conviction of belief.

On the following page is a sample zigzag form.

A SAMPLE ZIGZAG FORM
New Belief

Being happy and content increases my chances of having a positive impact on others.

__30_ % of conviction in this New Belief

RESPONSE: Realising that I am in a state of unhappiness and that it is unhelpful is the first step towards changing it.

RESPONSE: Nothing in life is guaranteed and there's no guarantee that doing all the "right things" (meditation, assertiveness, eating and sleeping well) will make me happy. But they *might*. The old belief is almost guaranteed to make me unhappy. Isn't the prospect of an uncertainly happy future better than a certainly miserable one?

RESPONSE: What could be worse than being tortured by your own mind's belief's that have in the past made me suicidal? As for the uncertainty, yeah it is an uncertain future. There will be ups and downs as there have always been. There will be [loss and disappointments]. But I will cope with this. Through letting go of this belief I will gain resilience to not just cope with them but learn from them. I cannot learn from suicide.

New rating of conviction __80__ %

ATTACK: Okay fine but I don't know how to be happy. I only know how to be angry. I'll never be happy.

ATTACK: But what if I fail? What if my attempts to be happy and content fail? I'll be left more unhappy because I tried.

ATTACK But I can't cope with that uncertainty. At least the misery and depression are familiar. Familiarity has its own kind of comfort. Think of Stockholm Syndrome and the phrase "The Devil You Know." What If I end up in a WORSE situation?

Quite often you will find that not only do the old, negative beliefs die hard, but that when they are vanquished, a new one will rise up to take its place. Again, that's okay. It's not a reason for discouragement or that you're not making progress. *Au contraire!* It actually means that you are progressing very well. Part of the process of REBT is to uncover deeper and deeper layers of belief, so that, eventually, you will find that you have dug down deep enough through the surface beliefs that you are now encountering the very deepest, core beliefs. At this point, you will know that you are finally working at the core of your being and that the changes you are making in how you process information about yourself, about others, your model of the world, and your tactics and strategies for getting needs met and nurturing yourself and others are lasting and permanent.

The Four Stages of Learning

Learning can be divided into four stages: unconscious incompetence; conscious incompetence; conscious competence; and unconscious competence.[3] Here is an example.

Unconscious incompetence: When I started out whitewater paddling it was in a canoe and I knew nothing about kayaking. I did not know that you could 'roll' a kayak. I didn't know what I didn't know.

Conscious incompetence: I was surprised to learn that if you flipped over and were upside down in the water, instead of coming out of your boat, you could use the paddle to roll yourself up. I still didn't know how to roll a kayak, but now I knew I didn't know.

Conscious competence: I developed conscious competence. I bought a book with instructions how to roll. At the side of a swimming pool I practised each step separately: set-up, sweep, hip-snap. Then I went to the middle of the pool, flipped upside down, put them together, and *voila*, I rolled up! Probably not on the first attempt. I don't remember. Now I knew how to do it, but I had to think about it, approach it systematically, and practise it.

Unconscious competence: one stage at a time, after lots of practice, I went to moving water, then to class 1 rapids, then class 2, classes 3, 4, and 5, where you didn't have time to think or prepare. You just had to do it. Automatic.

In the same way, REBT may be something your clients have never heard of or had any idea that it was possible, or desirable, to change how you feel about something by changing your belief about it. Now they know when you tell them. You have moved them from the first to the second stage. Next is developing conscious competence. This is where clients are liable to get discouraged. As one of the exercises in my REBT workbook puts it, 'I just can't understand this REBT. This just proves how worthless I am!' This phase can be daunting for clients. Persevere. It takes patience, practice, and persistence. Eventually they will get there. And of course, for you to teach them, you will need to know how to do it yourself.

Eventually REBT will become second nature, both for the client and the therapist. When it does, it will be running in the unconscious mind in procedural memory. It is a technique that begins with conscious intent and moves gradually into the unconscious.

Here is an example of using REBT with a client who uses a mixed A5–6/C3–4 strategy.

Bob and the Shroud of Shame

Bob was brought to me by his wife for fixing. Bob's wife, Sheila, had called to make an appointment for them as a couple. When we met, Sheila had numerous complaints: Bob's excessive drinking, his out of control anger, drunk or sober. He was not angry or violent towards her or their two children. He was violent towards strangers who had done something to anger him. This behaviour was exacerbated by his drinking. In addition, there was difficulty financially with their house they were renovating while living in it and with Bob's business failing.

They had a lot of work to do. There was no warmth between them. Sheila blamed Bob for all their problems. As I learned more about them, it was clear that wasn't true at all. Sheila bullied Bob into overextending himself to try to please her. Their house renovation was a big source of problems. Sending their girls to a posh private school was more than they could afford given their financial circumstances. Sheila was a professional, but in private practice she could work as little or as much as she liked. At that point, she was working very little. This was justified, in her mind, by the time she spent with their girls. Bob, on the other hand, was more of an absentee dad. He made the money and left the parenting to Sheila, so she did have a point. As we shall see, this arrangement exacerbated the dysfunctionality between them. Sheila took no responsibility for their financial straits; Bob took no responsibility for parenting or housework.

Bob's father had agreed to come help him with his business. His way of doing that was to stiff their suppliers. When I discussed this with Bob, he thought that was a brilliant way to go about it. I pointed out that the policy was, *per se*, self-defeating. By the time Bob realized this, it was too late to save Bob's business.

Almost immediately Sheila quit participating in therapy. She had delivered Bob to me for fixing, so apparently she thought that her part of it was done.

In his AAI, Bob identified five primary caregivers: his maternal grandmother who had taken him to raise while his mother, who was very young, pursued her career elsewhere; an aunt and uncle who helped to relieve the burden of raising a young child from their ageing mother; and then his mother and adoptive father. He never knew his biological father. During the early part of the interview, he became so distressed that I thought I was going to have to discontinue it. However, we carried on and the distress that had him near tears became anger as the interview went on.

Here is the last part of Bob's AAI:

> **Okay. So (sighs) [the sigh is sadness on my part. Pay attention to how you feel. This will give you great insight into the strategy] overall, what do you think you have learnt from your experiences as a child?**
> Self-reliance. Erm? … (3) I dunno.
> **Are there things that you are trying to do differently or the same with your children?**
> I am trying to be—spend more time with them
> **Are you?**
> You know, but sometimes Sh … I mean she is right in most things and you know. I see so many things in Lorrie that's the same as me, you know? Whereas Sheila controls it and nurtures it and cares for it, you know? And I just let her get on with it, as she is the best at doing it, you know?
> **Well we are at the end of the interview now, except for one last question, and that is—is there anything else that you want to add that you think is important in order to understand you—who you are today?**
> Just don't want to be a wasted life … (3) you know? Feel quite strongly about that (upset) … (3) you know, I've got—you know I almost feel as if I could be a use to humanity you know, that sounds a really—You know almost like fucking, like discover penicillin
> **Oh, yeah …**
> I've just got this—and yes, so I just don't want to be a wasted life.
> **Do you think you are?**
> At the moment, yeah. Lots of aspects make me feel like a wasted life, you know?
> **Okay. Anything else?**

I want to be a better dad and a husband.

Okay. Anything else?

Err? … (3) I want to start enjoying life again.

Okay … (4) anything else you want to add?

I want to be the person I know I can become. Not what people expect me to be.

Well, I believe going through this process will help you to do all of those things.

Okay.

Anything more?

Erm I would like to fucking finish something I started.

What?

I just said like—you know like, I have started a house but I haven't—what's the word I am looking for—I don't ever finish anything right because

ahh

What happens is that the more complex it is or whatever I get my mind into it and then when I get to a point where I know I can do it I lose interest and I can't get back onto it. Do you know what I mean?

mm

I mean it's like—yeah so that's quite frustrating for me because I get bored, do you know what I mean? and if my mind—as I say the more complex, the more difficult, I am always a good problem solver you know.

mm

but once I have solved it in my mind, I never finish anything, so then I get frustrated then, you know?

yes

It's—there is something—when I was—not when I was having difficulties, but I just gave up. It's my way of rebelling. When I was doing my 'O' levels and, you know, I was having trouble in maths and this that and the other, and erm, my mum goes, 'You have got'—to my dad—'you have got to help him. He is not doing very well at maths.' And my dad is like—I reckon it was three minutes—we sat down and we did all these high end maths equations: everything right. And he has got up and he has walked out the room and he goes to mum, 'He knows what he is doing. I can't teach him anything. He just needs to do it,' and that was it.

And did you know?

Yeah, I did. Yeah.

Okay.

But I had a mental block, you know? I put a mental block in my mind not to do it, you know what I mean? And now I can't get rid of that either, and I need to break it down. One other thing, one other thing: I used to have this recurring dream—recurring nightmare it was, not even a nightmare—if

I am in certain situations—where I am in one corner of the room, and it's pitch black and I can see every corner, every—and then there is just something in the room that gets bigger and bigger and bigger and I get smaller and smaller and smaller. And I had that recurring dream for years and years and years you know? And I would get smaller. As I said, it was pitch black. I can make everything out and then it was a matter, it was almost like me making myself get bigger to get out of the room but I have never got out of that room.

And when were you having that nightmare?

I had it from about six all the way up to about thirty six

Okay

As I said, I haven't ever gotten out of that room Charley—have never gotten out of that room.

Notice the present perfect tense when he says, 'And he has got up and he has walked out the room and he goes to mum.' This indicates that this event is still very current and very involving in Bob's emotions. He is re-experiencing it as he describes it, as if it is happening all over again.

Notice, too, the dichotomy: Bob knows the maths, so cognitively, factually, he gets it. What he doesn't have is *motivation* to do it. Emotions are what provide motivation and it is motivation that Bob needs in order to be successful. Both mom and dad seem oblivious to the obvious: if Bob knows cognitively how to do it, what is he lacking emotionally in order to be *motivated* to do it? By not doing it, Bob gains attention, nurturing.

Bob knows intuitively that there is something wrong, as reflected in what he goes on to share about his desire to be of benefit to others. His unconscious mind gives him an accurate analogy of the predicament in which he finds himself trapped in a dark room with no way out, with a 'presence' that gets bigger and bigger while he gets smaller and smaller.

He blames himself for his failure. Even though the information is there, metacognitively, he can't put it together. Despite his *desire* to be different, he lacks the motivation. His transcript is that of a depressed A+. There also seem to be elements of a C+ strategy from time to time, evidenced by his violence towards others and his explosive expression of anger, typically towards himself. However, that may be intrusions of negative affect or PTSD intrusions. There is also the maths that he is able to do but doesn't. This is C4, feigned helplessness. The depression is coded as a modifier. This means that it acts pervasively throughout the transcript to prevent integration and reorganization—and it consequently works that way in his life as well. The blend of strategies is not unusual when a child has to adapt to so many different caregivers. He had been operating out of A4, Compulsive Compliance; A6, Compulsive Self-reliance; and A7, Delusional Idealization where his father was concerned. He also, I would later discover, had elements of A5, Compulsive Promiscuity.

These were the challenges in the beginning of therapy. What motivation there was, in the form of anger in order to change things, got repressed by Bob, as he had learned to do in childhood. On one occasion, having been involved in an altercation between his mother and father, he wound up head-butting his father. These eruptions of violence often involved the police.

Therapy went on in a rather desultory manner. Although Bob wanted to get better, he saw himself as being unable to do anything differently, and he did not see any way out of his difficulties. This was perhaps the C4, feigned helplessness aspect. I have had quite a few clients now who went from A4/6 to C4. This is obviously a self-defeating alternation or blend of strategies. He worked hard and saw his primary duties as completing the renovation to the house, making money to keep his daughters in the private school, and paying off the creditors to whom his business owed money.

The house renovation had run afoul of the building inspectors. Following his father's advice, Bob had not gotten planning permission for the extension, and it exceeded allowable dimensions. This, combined with a lack of money, brought the renovations to a halt. Meantime, the business had failed. His wife asked him to move out, leading to separation and ultimately divorce.

With this, Bob completely stopped therapy. He saw no point in it. This is not unusual for someone with a depressed A+ strategy. This state of affairs carried on for a few months, but I couldn't get Bob out of my mind. I thought that he was selling himself short, that he had got a rotten deal, and that it was time that he did something for himself for a change. (Could this have been a response to a C6, Seductive strategy? If so it was intuited between us.) I emailed him. He protested that he couldn't afford my fee. That had been an issue before when he was struggling to make ends meet. I told him that it didn't matter, that we could make the fee something affordable for him.

I learned that Bob had become suicidal and had been hospitalized for a period of time. He had also gotten into legal trouble as a result of getting into fights. These two factors had convinced him that maybe he did need help after all, and the fee offer was one he couldn't refuse, so he came back. And that's when we got to doing serious work.

The areas of concern for Bob: foremost was work. While not necessarily the most important, it was the most pressing. He had his support payments to his wife and children which were 50% higher than the law would have required. He had agreed to them to assuage his guilt. He also felt honour bound to repay his business creditors, and he had his own living expenses. He felt guilty and ashamed for not spending time with his daughters and often let them down when he had promised to do something with him. In the background, as a constant factor, was his relationship with his family of origin. His mother was an appeaser, his adoptive father was a bully, and his half-sister was both entitled and indulged by his parents. All these factors contributed to his shame and guilt, grief and sadness.

Having closed his business, Bob turned to working for others. He was very good at what he did, as the A4 strategy meant that he was personally invested in always doing his best, even though he would sometimes be erratic due to emotional mis-management. He went through a series of jobs in which he was professionally successful but in which he was personally unfulfilled. Here is an example of what I mean.

The Contract: REBT in Action

In this session, Bob is dealing with shame. This kind of treatment had been a recurring theme in Bob's life, starting with the shame of rejection that he felt in childhood. The second dose of shame comes from his relationship with his daughters. As a result of his work in therapy, he wants to be closer to his daughters. But he is still approaching it from the avoidant's, 'What can I do for you?' perspective. The realization that he gets something from it too—the 'fix' as he calls it—seems to him unnatural.

Bob had emailed me over the weekend to say how upset he was about learning that a contract he had done the estimate for had been won by his company. He was upset rather than happy:

> Jim phoned me on something else, and he said 'Oh, well done. We won that big job. We won it on Tuesday.' This was on the Friday. And I said to him, 'I'm really pleased we won it, Jim, but actually, nobody has bothered even to phone me up and tell me, bearing in mind I have worked on it for six months.' I said, 'Actually, I am really fucked off. At best it's rude, but it just shows me that they don't value me.' And he was very apologetic and said, 'No, no that's wrong. They should have told you.' And in that split second, as I said, you know I just felt—I felt worthless. But I could feel it, I could

taste it, I could touch it you know? Fucking hell, what is the word I'm looking for? It was—I just can't describe it, it was almost—but in that split second I just felt it—felt just destroyed and erm, then basically shut down.

Bob goes from social interaction with Jim to the triple F when he believes
he has been ignored and slighted, and then into the flop mode (what
Porges calls 'death feigning'). I point out to him:

> **You didn't totally shut down. You said how you were feeling and what
> you thought about it.**
> Well, yeah I did. Yeah, which is a—which is a step forward which is
> good, erm.

Expressing feelings was something we had been working on consistently.
He then describes feeling 'hollow' for the rest of the day. I ask:

> **Have you used the term 'shame' for that?**
> No, I didn't use the word shame. It wasn't a feeling of shame, it was a feel-
> ing of worthlessness, you know? I just felt not valued, didn't feel valued.
> **Yeah, so that is the same thing as shame in my book.**
> Okay.
> **It's one thing to say, 'Well, they don't value me.' It's another for you
> to feel valueless yourself, and the good news is you are not feeling that
> way anymore, but you are reacting strongly when other people treat
> you that way.**
> Right okay.
> **And it sounds like your feelings were hurt? Yeah?**
> Oh, yeah! That was an understatement. I was talking about other projects
> with another contracts manager, and he went, 'I heard you won the big
> contract.' I went, 'Yes we did, but nobody fucking bothered telling me and
> he says, 'That says it all really, doesn't it?'
> **What do you think he meant by 'that says it all'?**
> There isn't good teamwork. We had a meeting on Thursday where we could
> air some grievances with our bosses, and the main thing that came up was
> communications: just don't communicate.
> **And when was this meeting?**
> This was on the Thursday.
> **Before the Friday?**
> Before the Friday, yeah.

Okay, so that is a great example of what they were talking about in the meeting.

We then discuss the company culture and how it is dysfunctional. Bob is still taking this failure to communicate personally. I want to use REBT to give him a different belief. First, I use an embedded NLP shift to move him from cause to effect:

Let's look at what you told yourself in order to create that feeling. We are not necessarily going to change it. How did you feel?
I felt like I said worthless. Like I said, everything I had done wasn't good enough. It just—it was a—it was erm a solid confirmation that I'm not even worth a phone call to say well done, you won a job.
Now, does that help you to deal with the situation?
No, it doesn't. No.
No, because it distorts the reality of it.
Yes.
And is it based on known facts and reality?
Well, it appears reality for me.
It's your reality?
Yes it appears reality to me.
Are you saying it feels that way?
Yes, it feels like reality
Okay. Let's take the feeling state out of that because feelings are *per se* subjective, okay?
Yeah.
Have you ever been to the IMax theatre? They have these movies where they are flying over the countryside and you are surrounded by the video, so it's a totally inclusive experience and so it feels like you are moving.
Yeah I have seen that, yeah.
But you are not. You are sitting on a seat and the seat is bolted to the floor. (chuckles)
Right, okay.
Okay?
Good. Yes.
How you are feeling and the reality can sometimes be two different things.
Right okay.

So, there is really strong evidence that it's *not* based on known facts and reality.

Okay?

You just shared the evidence with me that I am going to use. Do you remember what it was?

Err ...? No.

What about the meeting you had on Thursday?

(slowly) Yes ... Exactly ... [a pause, I can tell from his eye movements he is thinking] Yeah? ... [still thinking] Oh, I see what you mean. Yeah. Yeah!

That meeting was evidence, that was acknowledgement: 'We have a problem with communication in this company.'

Right, okay, yeah. Basically yeah and it was flagged up. You know, we made light of it and jokes about it a couple of times, but then the following day that happens and erm, as I said, you know my, my self-confidence, my self-esteem is quite low at the moment and it just, sort of—it was very fragile and that just broke it, really badly you know?

I really want to focus on the REBT approach to what you were telling yourself about that event

Yes, okay.

I want to really emphasize how good it is. I think it's a real change. Do you think it's a change that you spoke up and said something at all?

Erm I think it is a change, erm yes, if I look at it now it was a change and it was an instant reaction. It wasn't something that erm ... Yeah, I instantly knew it was wrong and I instantly knew how it made me feel.

This is a good example of how changes take place spontaneously when the unconscious mind has been re-programmed. He is still struggling how to express negative feelings in a constructive way. We are well into his zone of proximal development (ZPD). I reinforce to Bob that the problem is with his company, not with himself. He then starts to 'should' on himself by saying he 'should' have realized that.

Stop, stop, stop! I don't want to make that a 'should' either, because if you say, 'Well, I *should* have done that,' now you are just shaming yourself!

Yeah, I see what you mean. Yeah.

You were still interpreting it through that old lens of, 'I'm the one at fault here. I'm the one who is wrong here. How can I make this be my fault? Well, I'll just make it be about them not valuing me. Same old story.'

Yeah.

> 'Here I am, sunk deep in my shame again. Oh fuck, things will always
> be this way. I'll never be, blah blah blah ...' and all those things right
> off that page in the REBT workbook about the hot links—the things
> that lead to negative feelings. You know what I mean?
> Okay.

We discuss this some more, then Bob moves on to talking about the relationship with his daughters. There is linkage here, between the topics, and
the link is shame:

> Saturday it was Peggy's sixteenth birthday, so I went round there in the
> morning, give her a card, give her some money and erm, some flowers and
> a cake, erm and saw her in the morning, erm and—erm ... (6) erm I just, it,
> what—it wasn't anything to do with Sheila or the house or anything like
> that, I just felt that I only ever needed to be there for about forty five min-
> utes. I felt ... it's almost like erm ... you know like erm ... it was almost like
> you know I just needed that fix to see the children, actually, happy to leave
> you know, so once I had had my fix I was happy to leave, you know? I inter-
> acted with them, I interacted with them to a level that I felt comfortable at,
> and then, you know, then I let them get on their way and I, I left.

This is a put-down of himself. He considers it wrong to get joy from the
relationship with his children. He is unable just to enjoy their relationship,
spending time together. Like other A+ strategists, he is comfortable doing
things, giving them money or gifts, but not just being with them.

> **Well so what do you think about that and how do you feel about it?**
> Erm, I think there is a realisation that erm, you know four years is a long
> time. They have done a lot of growing up and I haven't been able to be
> there for them in the way I want, or been, or what they needed. Erm, I
> realise that erm, I am only a very small part of their life at the moment, and
> I realised that it's not going to be, you know, you know I am not going to
> win father of the year and erm there is a lot of—I can't force myself on them,
> you know? I can't force my time on them and it is probably going to be a
> very long journey to win a lot more trust back.
> **Well I think so, I think that's a realistic assessment of it.**
> Yeah. I mean Sunday Carol said, 'You know, it's not going to be a perfect
> relationship, or, you know, a very close relationship for some time. You have
> got to rebuild that trust and they've got to let their barriers down and let
> you back into their lives.'
> **And do they have a reason to do that?**

Erm—what to—to let me back in?
Yeah. I mean are you knocking on the door saying I want back in?
Erm, no. I am not really, no. I'm—what's the word I am looking for? I am scared to do that Charley.
What's the fear about? What are you afraid of?
The fear of rejection, the fear that they are not going to let me back in their lives the way I want to be back in their lives.
The way you want to be?
Yeah the way I want to be, erm fear that erm, if I push them too hard I will push them away too hard and hurt them.
Could be.
They are the two basic fears. And also there is a fear deep down that, you know—that, there are other male figures in their lives that would be more important to them when I have been growing up.

Notice the use of 'I' instead of 'they,' above. This is confusion of person again, as we saw with Rehan. It is common in the AAIs and speech of high numbered A and C strategies. I interpret this to be an indication that Bob's unconscious mind is merging his own experience growing up, when his father wasn't there for *him*: hence the misuse of 'I'—with the experience of *them*: his daughters growing up when he was not there for them. This is a source of guilt and shame, and it is because this emotional theme is an outgrowth and a continuation of his origins of his own guilt and shame that the unconscious mind confuses the two. It is also the fact that he is 'growing up' in his efforts to become a more responsible parent and also speaking up for himself at work. This is good progress that Bob is able to articulate his fear and his thoughts about why he has that fear. There is no point trying to sugar-coat the reality:

And that maybe makes it sting a little bit more, when you think, 'Well my dad wasn't a good father to me, but look at me, you know, I haven't been a good father to my girls.'
No.
So I think that's where ultimately forgiveness is required all around, you know?
Yeah.
I find it interesting that equation of shame and guilt versus grief and loss. I feel grief about what I did not get from my father: the loss.
Yeah.
And at the same time
I feel shame for what I am not giving out.

I noticed in the treatment centre long ago the guilt=grief equation: that when people who have either unresolved, it is usually balanced by an equal measure of the other. I know that Bob is with me and we have good rapport, because he completed my thought with 'I feel shame for what I am not giving out.' Bob takes the lead:

> **That's right. So I think part of your fear is, 'Well … if they get to know the real me, they won't like me.'**
> Yeah when you look at it like that…
> **What happens if you look at it like that?**
> Yeah, it's quite—err, yeah it's just a different way of looking at things…
> **It is…**
> Err, erm, quite helpful way of looking at it, Charley, in all honesty.
> **Well I was just going to ask—is that helpful to you? To look at it that way?**
> It is, it is. I mean I think I was saying or I was going to say to you earlier that, like—today I woke up and I almost look forward to, to—erm, I look forward to the day, shall we say, you know?
> **Really? Good!**
> I woke up and I said to Tanya this morning, 'I have probably felt as good this morning as I have done you know for—quite some time, really.' We took the dog out for a walk. She's got a dog and I realised you know I've missed, I miss my dog and I miss that responsibility and interaction with animals you know and it's just—I used to think, 'Oh well, you know I will never have another dog again.' But now I think, 'Well you know, if I get into a long term relationship with a bit of stability I will have a dog again,' that sort of—that sort of mindset you know. So I am much more looking forward than looking back.

Not long after this, Bob resumed work for himself. His business is doing well and growing quickly, thanks in part to his new romantic partner, a successful business-woman herself, who is helping him run his company and also helping him in his relationships.

Their relationship is developing in a typical A and C pattern. Whether they will be able to reconcile these differences and become more balanced and secure in their relationship remains to be determined.

This completes the REBT process. However, there is another use that we can put the new belief that gives us an effective emotional response (the E part of the ABCDE acronym) to use: we can make it into an affirmation.

NOTES

1. https://www.psychologytoday.com/gb/blog/the-three-minute-therapist/201703/5-major-differences-between-rebt-cbt.
2. Notarius, C., & Markman, H. (1993). *We can work it out: Making sense of marital conflict.* Putnam Adult. Gottman, J. (2018). *The seven principles for making marriage work.* Hachette UK. Driver, J., Tabares, A., Shapiro, A., Nahm, E. Y., & Gottman, J. M. (2003). Interactional patterns in marital success and failure: Gottman laboratory studies.
3. DePhillips, F. A., Berliner, W. M., & Cribben, J. J. (1960). *Management of Training Programs.* Homewood, Illinois: Bob D. Irwin.

CHAPTER 6

Reprogramming the Unconscious Mind

The intention of ACT is to reprogramme the unconscious mind. Even though the previous two chapters dealt with tools for working with the conscious mind, the real power is with the unconscious mind. Our cognitive analysis of the discourse in the AAI is based on our understanding gained through a conscious mind process. Likewise, when we have outcomes that we don't like, we can consciously use REBT to examine whether or not beliefs are rational. Then we can consciously reprogramme them. The first method that I present is the use of affirmations.

AFFIRMATIONS

Some writers in the pop psychology field assert that affirmations don't work. I can affirm that they do. If they haven't worked for you in the past, then these instructions will help you to make then work. I will tell you the secret in a bit. First, let's pick up with the 'Effective' new belief from REBT from the previous chapter. This new belief can be made into an affirmation. This will help to get it programmed into the mind so that it becomes the new default belief. Remember that we having been giving ourselves 'defamations' for years. Don't be surprised if the affirmation takes a while.

C. Shults, *Attachment Centred Therapy*, Palgrave Texts in Counselling and Psychotherapy, https://doi.org/10.1007/978-3-031-60851-3_6

The New Belief as Affirmation

I suggest writing the new belief/affirmation on an A4 sheet of paper, quite large and bold, or however you like it, and taping it to your mirror. That way, every time you look in the mirror, you will be reminded of your affirmation. Each day, morning and evening, while awakening and before going to bed, look yourself in the eye and repeat your affirmation three times. That's all there is to it. You will be amazed when, after a few days, weeks, or months, you will begin to make this your default state of mind, rather than the old default.

Oh, but wait! You say you've tried that, and it doesn't work? In fact, you feel more of a fraud because you are telling yourself something that you *know*, in the core of your being is untrue? This introduces the barf factor.

Why Some People Think They Don't Work: The Barf Factor

This is that feeling that you get when you try to do the affirmation and feel sick to your stomach, awkward, embarrassed, even ashamed. When you try to affirm something that is opposite to what has been your established way of thinking and feeling about yourself, it feels unnatural, false, wimpish, whiny, or whatever impression you have been pre-programmed to feel about yourself when you try to be kind to yourself.

When some people say to themselves, 'I am a good and worthy person,' then they might hear another voice inside that says, *'NO BY GOD YOU'RE NOT! YOU'RE SCUM, YOU LITTLE SHIT, AND YOU NEVER WILL BE WORTH A DAMN!'*

Ouch! Nobody wants to invite that kind of wrath.

Maybe the voice is different. Maybe it says, quietly, smugly, 'Now, you know that's not true—you little liar.' Either way, it negates what you just tried to affirm.

So, if you really don't believe it, then don't try to lie to yourself. Instead, don't fight the problem, seek the solution. Simply modify the affirmation with the six magic words.

The Six Magic Words: 'I Would Like to Believe That'

Make it, '*I would like to believe that* I am a good and worthy person.' Amazingly, that seems to silence the critic *almost* every time. Why? Because it is the truth. You *would* like to believe it, if only you could. A part of you desires to be better than you are in some way, or you would not be reading this now. You would not be in therapy or be a therapist yourself (or both). You would not be trying as hard as you can to do better, to have better relationships, to be more at peace with yourself and your life.

Sometimes, even this trick doesn't work. That was the case with Bob. I had enquired if he was doing the affirmations. He said that he was, but that they weren't working. I asked him to tell me what his experience was. He assured me that he was doing them as suggested. I asked him what happened immediately afterwards.

'Well,' he said, 'I go back to hating myself and tell myself what a fucking idiot I am!'

Stop it! Cancel, Cancel! Affirmation!

Once you begin using the affirmations, you will find that the old defamations are still in there, ready to make an appearance anytime there is an opportunity. When you find yourself defaming yourself once again, then here is a corrective technique. First, internally shout to yourself, '**STOP IT!**' Get angry at this voice in your head and direct that angry energy towards refuting it. Next, follow this command with another command: 'Cancel, Cancel!' A simple and straightforward instruction by your conscious mind to cancel the previous negative command or statement. This works to counter-condition the automatic negativity by stopping it and cancelling it. As a general rule it is better to say what you want, not what you don't want. But in a situation where you have automatically and routinely defamed yourself, you need to make a big deal about refuting it when you catch yourself doing it.

BREATH WORK: PRANAYAMA

Pranayama is the yogic science of breath.[1] A recent exposition is *Breath: A Scientific Approach to a Lost Art* by James Nestor.[2] (Contrary to the subtitle, it has never been 'lost.') And then there is Wim Hof who is a current YouTube star with his breathing accomplishments. Amazing things can be done through the breath and meditation. In *Breath*, Nestor describes Swami Rama voluntarily 'stopping' his heart for 17 seconds. Don't worry. You're not going to have to learn to do that! The point is that breath work and mind control are keys to mastering one's physiology.

Breath work is important for a number of reasons. The primary benefit of breathwork, the first step of which needs to be to learn to breathe properly, deeply and calmly, is to be able to calm and soothe the nervous system. When someone is anxious and distressed, angry, upset, any kind of difficult emotional state, then to focus on the breath in a calming way is beneficial. It can also be used for energizing, for those who might be depressed, and in many other ways. What we are interested in here is the way to maintain balance within the voluntary and autonomic nervous systems, and consequently the enteric nervous system.

Based on my experience combined with research, such as Porges' polyvagal theory,[3] it is my belief that there are three systems or levels of arousal to the central nervous system. The first is the social interaction level. This is where things are nice and calm, we can interact easily with others. Next is the triple F: freeze, fight, flight. Some models consider this to be simply fight or flight. But I've been there. If you are suddenly confronted with danger—a predator, a man with a gun pointed at you—your first instinct is likely going to be to freeze. This is often preceded by a sharp intake of breath and then breath cessation while in the freeze state. It is easy to imagine how this has great evolutionary advantage. If you are suddenly surprised by a predator or an enemy in proximity, but they haven't discovered your presence yet, then holding the breath can save your life. It will help prevent detection. To breathe will produce movement, sound, smell. Any of these could give away your presence and location. As you freeze in position and hold your breath, your mind is racing. What is my best option here? Remain frozen? I'm going to have to breath eventually. But it must be very slow and controlled. What if I run? Can I get away? Or is that only going to be turning my back on my enemy or the predator? Do I fight? If they haven't detected me yet I will have the advantage of surprise. If I do start running or fighting, then my breath is going to be supercharged.

But let's say the predator grabs me. Now I'm in the tigers jaws, gripped by its teeth. Am I going to be 'frozen?' Hell no. Because that lets the predator know that *I am alive and alert!* My predator is not going to like that and is going to take steps to curtail both. What I am going to do is what Porges calls death feigning. That term I agree with. We do feign death, whether I am the soldier in the tiger's mouth, the chipmunk that the cat brought in, or the fawn in the 'deer protects her fawn' video.[4] We go flop. Totally limp, non-resistant. To call this 'freeze' is to misapply the word. Freeze implies rigidity. Flop is the opposite.

Deep Breathing—the Deep Breath

Deep breath in pranayama means a breath that goes to the deepest part of the lungs. It does not mean a *full* or *complete* breath which means the three parts of the breath together: deep, middle, and upper. When the deep breath is being used, the abdomen goes in when the breath goes out and it goes out when the breath goes in. A good way to really get the feel of this movement, if you aren't already aware of it, is to lie down on your back and get comfortable. Place one hand on your abdomen between the solar plexus (that area where the two sides of the ribs meet at the bottom of the sternum) and the navel, or belly button. You will then feel the rise and fall of your hand as you breath in and then out. If you are not feeling this, then you aren't relaxed enough yet. So, focus on your breathing and slow it down until you do. No effort is required to breath this way, so if you are 'trying' to do it, don't: just lie there and observe your hand going up and down. When you are totally relaxed, you will naturally breathe this way.

After you have gotten used to this feeling, try sitting up in whatever way is most comfortable for you so that you can retain your feeling of relaxation as much as possible and simply carry on with the deep breathing.

The Middle Breath

Now let's identify the middle and upper breaths to continue our exploration of pranayama. The middle breath is roughly the rib cage area. You can identify this breath by continuing to sit upright (it will be good if you can observe yourself in a mirror as you do this so that you can get immediate visual feedback). Place a hand on each side of your rib cage. Keep the rest of your body still, including the abdominal muscles which produce the deep breath, and breath into the chest. You should see your hands going out to the side and then back towards the middle as your rib cage, or thorax, expands and contracts with each breath in and out. Again, when the breath goes in, the ribs go out, and vice versa. If you practise with this kind of breathing, you will notice that it takes much more energy than deep breathing and creates a state of tension in the body because you have to actively use muscles to expand the chest and draw in the air. Once you have established this, now try your deep breathing again, and notice how much easier it is than chest, or middle, breathing. This is because, in order to breath from the abdomen, all we have to do is relax: relax the diaphragm—just let go—and the air automatically rushes in to fill the vacuum created. After inhalation, simply relax again, and you will find that the abdominal wall automatically moves inward forcing the air out. Relax the abdomen again, and the next breath flows in, and so on.

The Upper Breath

Now let's go to the upper breath. If you suffer from anxiety, and if you looked at yourself in the mirror while you were breathing in the earlier part of this exercise, you may have noticed that your shoulders lifted with each breath. If you were breathing deep or middle, you would not have noticed this. Many people who suffer from anxiety hold their bodies in a rigid frame, muscles tense in the torso, and unconsciously breathe by lifting the shoulders. This is the hardest job of breathing there is. It requires not only the involvement of the shoulder and neck muscles, where tension is apt to accumulate anyway, but it is also fighting the force of gravity by lifting a part of the body up! Again, if you want to experience how hard this is, keep the abdominal wall still, keep the rib cage from expanding laterally (if you leave your hands on the side of the rib cage you can easily tell whether or not you are involving this middle breath), and breath only by lifting the shoulders. If you are someone who is more or less naturally relaxed and instinctively breathing more or less correctly, then you will find that this type of breathing is very unnatural and tiring, and you will begin to feel more tense and anxious as you do it.

If, on the other hand, this way of breathing *is your default way of breathing*, then I will be very surprised if you do not suffer from generalized anxiety disorder. If anxiety is an issue for you, check your breathing. I have yet to encounter anyone who suffered from chronic anxiety who didn't breathe this way.

Whether this is cause or effect is debatable, because when we are anxious about something, we are likely to tense our bodies automatically. Anxiety is fear, after all, about what is about to happen. When we feel fear, our bodies tend to go rigid, and some people have a rather rigid muscular/skeletal system that has been referred to as 'body armour.' Indeed, this rigidity and tenseness of muscles is probably the body's natural response, wired in through evolution, to help us survive attacks and accidents.

The Full Breath

But let's get back to breathing correctly. If you have been following along with this, then you have identified the three parts of the breath and where and how they are located in your body. You have experimented with how each feels in the body and the mood induced in the mind. Now we can put them together to take a full, or complete, breath. To do this, simply go back to your deep breathing. On the next inhalation, after the deep breath comes in and the abdomen goes out, simply continue drawing in air and you will notice that your rib cage lifts and expands as additional air rushes in and *is supported by* the deep breath. Now, continue to draw in the last bit of air until the lungs are completely full, and you will notice that the shoulders naturally rise without much effort as this upper breath fills the lungs, expanding them, and completes the intake cycle. Do this several times and notice how easily the rib cage expands and the shoulders lift, because each is supported by the preceding level. When you are ready to exhale, just let go and the air goes out in reverse order. Simple.

Normally, we don't do the full breath, as that much volume of air exchange isn't needed. But we ought to always use the deep breath as that is the way to most effectively oxygenate the blood, it uses the least energy, and it keeps us relatively relaxed.

If you are accustomed to breathing wrongly—as many of us are—then it will take a bit of time and training to make the deep breath your default, and this is where mindfulness comes in: simply being mindful, or aware, of your breath, one breath at a time, and consciously choosing to use the deep breath.

When we are alarmed—when our triple F kicks in—our heartrate accelerates, our breathing becomes rapid and shallow, our muscles tense and pre-stress by shaking and trembling, we may feel a flushing sensation over our bodies, and so on. If we are really threatened, our breathing may actually stop. Our digestion ceases as energy is diverted to muscles for fight or flight, and we feel 'a knot in the gut.' There may be, in extreme cases, voiding. This is the unconscious mind, our autonomic sympathetic nervous system, getting ready to deal with danger.

If you have trained your unconscious mind, then it will be looking to your executive function for *what* to do but not *how* to do it. The unconscious is much faster and much more powerful and intuitive than your executive could ever be. We've already looked at this phenomenon of rolling a kayak. At my best, if I flipped in whitewater, I was quickly back up without having to think about it. It was automatic. Martial artists and race car drivers, to mention just a few, practise a great deal to master these skills so that their unconscious mind knows what to do without the executive having to delay the process to issue a command.

But this doesn't always work. If you are at work, your co-worker is likely not your enemy, and so killing him or her, or even giving them a sound drubbing, would be contraindicated. Even worse, what about the person with whom you share a bed at night? Do you really want to throttle them? Or is it your unconscious misinterpreting things and over-reacting into the triple F, or the dread death feigning of the Flop mode?

What breathwork allows us to do is to learn to use the deep breath to calm the mind. Of all the physiological mechanisms triggered by the triple F, the breath is the one that we can easily learn to control, and when we calm and slow the breath, then the heartrate, muscle tone, and other physiological responses follow suit, calming the mind and body. This is the first and most physiologically rewarding aspect of breathwork.

Second, because your breath is controlled largely by your unconscious mind until you become mindful of it, and then it can be controlled by the conscious mind, controlling the breath becomes a way of integrating the conscious and unconscious aspects of mind. When you are controlling your breath with the conscious mind, the unconscious mind is monitoring what is going on and is ready to step in should the need arise.

We can think of the mind as being composed of three functions that have tremendous overlap. First is the deep unconscious, the life support system that is all powerful. This I analogize to the elephant. There is some manipulation that can be done via the conscious mind. For example, the siddha yogis who practise meditation in regular clothing outside in the freezing weather of the Himalayas. Next is the pre-conscious, or limbic system, that can be programmed, to some extent, by doing things like learning to ride a bicycle, roll a kayak, having an internalized map of the streets of London, performing surgery. This we can think of as the monkey mind, that can be chattering, jabbering, hopping about, and distracting us. Our conscious mind, or executive function, is like the mahout who decides, okay, I'm going to meditate now. That is what happens when we, the mahout, connect *directly* to the elephant through the breath that allows us to slip into the state called meditation.

MEDITATION

I think many people who try meditation are put off because they misunderstand what it is, become frustrated, and decide that they can't possibly do it. So what is intended to be a positive experience becomes another reason to put oneself down. Meditation is quite simple. Maybe that is what makes it so hard! Here is how to do it:

1. Find a quiet place and make yourself comfortable.
2. Breathe deeply, starting with three full breaths, then just breath naturally.
3. Continue watching the breath.

Done that? Good. You were meditating. When you get really good at it, you can skip step one. And then step two.

'But wait,' you say. 'It's not that easy!'

I didn't say it was going to be easy. I said it was simple. This is where discipline and practice come in. Your conscious mind is not used to having nothing to worry about, think about, or do. So, you have to train it. Really, it is the monkey mind, the preconscious or limbic system, that you are training. Like a wilful child, your monkey mind is going to keep tugging at the shirtsleeve of your consciousness trying to get your attention. Be a kind parent to yourself and patiently listen, or watch, as the distraction plays itself out. Then gently return your awareness to your breath. Just keep doing this. Slow, relaxed breathing tells the mind, through physiological messaging, to slow down and relax. This bypasses the monkey mind. The monkey mind eventually grows extremely bored and falls asleep, and then the conscious and unconscious can merge. If you want more, the best meditation book I know of is Lawrence LeShan, *How to Meditate*.[5]

When REBT is combined with meditation, the two together can be very powerful. Once the REBT process is learned, it is quite simple to apply it during the contemplation phase of meditation. As you observe your thoughts and feelings, become a 'witness' and simply watch them as they roll by, imagine that you are sitting on a hillside overlooking a pleasant valley on a warm, sunny day. Imagine the thoughts and feelings as shadows that clouds make as they pass over a sunlit valley and then disappear.

If a thought or feeling captures your mind momentarily, as soon as you realize that your awareness has wandered from your breath, simply bring it back. Don't worry about how or why it wandered. Just gently bring it back as you would a small child. If you find that some of these thoughts or feelings are persistently returning, or if it is something that really grabs your attention, such as a memory of abuse that had previously been repressed, then you need to make a mental or physical note to deal with that. You can literally make notes, if you desire, during meditation. Simply rise to a minimal level necessary for making the note, then return to the deeper level of meditation. That will often help to put persistent worries to one side.

The yogis have helpfully divided meditation into four steps. The first it to withdraw awareness from the senses and to focus one's awareness on a single point. That is why we find a quiet place where we can be comfortable. There are many ways to do this. I prefer to keep it simple and focus on the breath. Second is contemplation in which we think about things. I typically focus on a chakra meditation. We might also contemplate the distractions that our monkey mind keeps presenting to us. It is during this phase that we might find ourselves having a random thought about something at work and who said what to whom winding up with you telling the boss they can take this job and shove it! Oh dear. And then you remember you're supposed to be meditating. Oh well, just bring your awareness back to your breath. Rinse and repeat. Let go of whatever it was, breathe deep, and relax. Eventually, when you have trained the mind sufficiently, you will fall into meditation. And eventually, when you have fallen into meditation enough, you will reach samadhi. Then you will experience knowledge, existence, bliss: satchitananda.

But don't hold your breath!

NLP, HYPNOTHERAPY, AND TIME LINE THERAPY®

It is unfortunate that NLP is so polarizing. On the one hand are its advocates who exaggerate its efficacy, and on the other are its detractors who believe that it is humbug for the weak-minded. I think it is a useful tool that, properly understood and utilized, can be a very effective intervention and can also help to provide a sound basis for more traditional forms of therapy by understanding how the mind works, conscious, pre-conscious, and unconscious (mahout, monkey, elephant).

Rapport

Perhaps the most useful skill is rapport building. It is the only form of therapy that I have encountered that teaches you how to identify rapport and create and maintain rapport, yet rapport is key to the therapeutic relationship. Rapport is what we can think of as 'being in sync' with the other person. In Bob's story earlier you saw an example of good rapport. The evidence is that he often completed my thoughts, even when the points that I am making, if done without rapport, could be offensive and threatening to the relationship.

You are influencing your clients more than you probably realize from the first moment of contact. Your unconscious mind is taking in information, processing it, and presenting your conscious mind with thoughts, feelings, and impressions from the get-go. The client is likewise forming an impression of you. Are you kind, cruel, frightening, friendly, helpful, altruistic, self-seeking, judgemental? Your facial expression, rate and location of breath, tone of voice, posture, gestures, in short, everything about you is giving the client an impression.

There are things that you can do to improve rapport and create trust, and there are things you can do that will alienate and create mistrust. Knowing the difference can determine the outcome of therapy even before you start. Any good NLP book will tell you how to do this, and any good NLP training course will give you opportunities to practise.

Programming

Beyond rapport, NLP gives a useful description of the unconscious mind, how it operates, and makes suggestions for how to use that information to advantage. The basic premise is simple: we have experiences from the past to which we respond by 'learning' from them; we then draw on those experiences, *the most important and influential of which are deeply buried and not consciously accessible,* in knowing how to respond to here and now situations; based on this information we then make 'if/then' or causal predictions about the outcomes of our behaviour; finally, we form a plan, or what the DMM calls a 'dispositional representation,' and proceed to execute it. We call this entire process a 'program,' hence the 'programming' in the name. This programme is embedded in neurology via the 'language' that we use, hence the 'neurolinguistics' in the name. This is

consistent with the DMM and REBT. The DMM would call these programmes 'procedural memory' or 'how to do something.'

Visual Acuity

Another valuable skill is visual acuity. NLP will give you training in how to
notice shifts in physiology that indicate internal changes. Eye movements
(on which Eye Movement Desensitization and Reprogramming (EMDR)
is based) are the most obvious and misunderstood visual cues. Others are
skin tone, flushing, blanching, tumescence, and I imagine there are others
that I haven't listed here. Breathing is one of them. Not only is the rate of
breath significant, but the location of the breath is of equal if not more
importance. That is covered in the pranayama section. Pulse is another. A
story about Milton Erickson is that he could tell that a client had gone
into trance by the pulse he could see in a vein on her ankle.

ERICKSONIAN HYPNOTHERAPY

Another benefit of NLP is learning about the language patterns of Milton
Erickson.[6] Erikson embedded his hypnosis conversationally, naturally. You
will learn to use trance states, both those that you induce and those that
occur naturally. We go in and out of trance naturally. Meditation is an
adjunct of this. NLP techniques can seem gimmicky, granted. And they
are. Gimmicks work. I have gravitated away from using those techniques.
The importance is in learning *how* they work and the principles they use.
Then you can incorporate those techniques in your work in a naturalistic
manner, *a la* Erickson. This involves 'utilization,' meaning that whatever
happens in the situation can be utilized and incorporated into the therapeutic process. I will use these language patterns throughout the examples
that I give.

TIME LINE THERAPY®

Time Line Therapy® (TLT) is the *piece de resistance* of NLP. It utilizes the
realm beyond time and space, or what Jung called 'the collective unconscious,' in Vedantic philosophy 'the akasha,' to make changes rapidly and
give new meaning to historical events. When we 're-member,' the one
member of the recollection that we *can* change is the meaning that we
give to it. This meaning is a new belief that is positive, about the self, and

future-oriented. This allows the client to re-experience the event with a sense of efficacy and a new meaning that the unconscious mind can apply to all such events. When I first heard about TLT, I thought that it sounded too good to be true. (You may think so, too!) But then I remembered a couple of experiences that I had that supported the idea: Adlerian Life Style Analysis and Tina and the Teacup.

Adlerian Life Style Analysis

Alfred Adler had the same idea.[7] By going back to the earliest memories that one had, new and more useful beliefs can be created about that event using one's adult experiences. After all, when these events occurred in infancy or early childhood, we had little if any understanding cognitively of what was going on. The new beliefs would then allow the client to make sweeping changes in their lives.

I set out to use this new technique that emphasized getting to the earliest memories associated with a particular emotion and examining the learning from it, then creating a new and more effective learning. It worked. But not well enough. That is, sometimes we could get really good results, but more often than not, the result was not outstanding. As a result, I decided to abandon that technique. But I remembered it when I was trying to decide about whether to take the TLT course.

Tina and the Tea Cup

I also remembered an event with a client where this effect had occurred spontaneously. Tina came to see me because she had trouble with anger: she couldn't express it. She was a doormat for others. Tina had worked out that the problem went back to her mother and we had been working on numerous events from childhood where she knew that she had needed to be able to use her anger to stand up for herself but had been unable to do so. The problem affected all areas of her life, especially in her career.

Then one day she came in and asked, 'Is it possible to have a memory that you have never had before, but you know that is a memory of a real event and not something made up?' I replied that it was, and enquired if she had such a memory.

'Yes,' she said. 'I was helping my mother clean out the basement in our house that I grew up in. We were going through boxes to decide what to keep and what to get rid of. I opened one of the boxes and inside was a set of china dishes that I hadn't seen since childhood. I picked up one of the delicate china teacups and held it up to the light, and that is when this memory came rushing back. It was as if a curtain had parted to reveal a scene on a stage.'

'My goodness,' I said, 'tell me about it.'

'My mother had been entertaining some of her friends, and when the tea party was over, I was helping her to clean up, the way little girls will do. I put one of the tea cups into the dish washer, and mother didn't see it. She ran the dishwasher, and when she opened it, she saw the tea cup, cracked. This was heirloom china that had been passed down from mother to daughter in her family, and when she saw the broken tea cup, she went berserk. She yelled at me, called me stupid, and banished me from the kitchen. She never let me help her again. And she put the set of china away, in that box, never to be seen until I opened it.'

'Oh dear,' I said. 'That was quite an over-reaction by mom.'

'Really?' she asked.

'Really,' I replied. I then asked her how she had felt. Ashamed, embarrassed, guilty, and afraid, she answered. I pointed out that it wasn't her fault that the cup had gotten broken. She disagreed and said that it was her fault: she had put the tea cup in the dishwasher. I acknowledged that was true, but pointed out to her that she had no way of knowing it wasn't okay to do that. It was mom's fault because she had been inattentive to what Tina was doing. We spent the entire session with the ins and outs of what had gone wrong and what might have happened instead. When Tina left, I thought that she had accepted my interpretation of events and that it hadn't been her fault, but rather mom's, and that mom had wrongly blamed her to avoid taking responsibility herself.

The next week Tina came in. 'What shall we work on today? Shall we work on more of these events when you felt angry with mom but couldn't express it?' I enquired. She thought for a long while.

'I don't need to work on any of those anymore,' she said.

I was surprised. Tina was very good at taking the initiative in working on her issues so I did not attribute her assertion to denial. 'Really? Why not?' I asked.

'Well, after I left here last week, I thought about what you had said, what had gone on between my mom and me, and then all the other times when she had treated me the same way and I had just taken it. And I realized, the way I had responded on those later times were based on what had happened in that first event with the teacup. And I realized that how I had dealt with anger ever since had been based on how she treated me about the teacup. It wasn't my fault. She was blaming me, but it wasn't my fault. Then I knew that it was okay for me to be angry and assert myself when someone mistreated me. And when I thought about the other events, the anger and resentment wasn't there anymore. It was gone.'

I was astonished. I had never heard of that before. But I remembered the Adlerian Life-Style analysis seminar. 'Wow,' I thought, 'if I could do that with all my clients, wouldn't that be something?'

It Damn Works!

So, here was Tad James offering to sell me a set of audio tapes that would teach me how to do this. I was still sceptical, but here was the kicker: a one-year money back guarantee if I wasn't satisfied. I took the plunge, bought the tapes, listened to them, and decided to give it a try with one of my clients.

She was a rough around the edges farmer. No nonsense, and I knew if it wasn't to her liking she would let me know. We did the first session with anger and resentment. Doing the tests, it seemed to work. She would see how it went for a week and let me know.

A week later, she began. 'You know that shit we did last week?' 'Yes?' I replied. 'It damn,' here she paused, raised one hand, and slapped it down on her knee, 'works!'

Whew. I breathed a sigh of relief. I have used TLT since. I also realized why the Adlerian Life-Style analysis technique had been so hit or miss: it is essential to get back to the first event for that particular tranche of emotions in order to get rid of the emotions from the past completely. With Tina and the teacup, we just got lucky. She happened upon a physical trigger for a repressed memory. The Adlerian technique relied on asking the client to access their memory using the conscious mind. Only rarely could the person remember what the first event was because that event is usually *prior* to conscious memory formation. And even when it is remembered consciously, its significance is not apparent.

TLT relies on gleaning information from the unconscious mind about the first event. That is why it is predictably reliable at getting rid of traumas, phobias, and negative emotions from the past.

The Lights Are Bright

Here is an example. Freda had been plagued with anxiety all her life. She said that she had been raped three times, in each case by someone she knew and had chosen to be with. I said that I thought that she was like the villagers in the story of the little boy who cried wolf. Her anxiety had been raising the alarm so consistently that she had learned to ignore it; hence, she could not distinguish between genuine threat and benign situations. She reckoned that was probably accurate. Regardless, she agreed with doing TLT to get rid of whatever negative feelings from the past were causing the problem.

TLT was still fairly new to me at the time, so when we finished the procedure, I enquired what it was about the first event, which for her was immediately after birth, that had been frightening.

'The lights were bright, I was cold, and I could move my arms and legs,' she said. I thought that was very interesting. She had just emerged from a warm, dark womb where her movements would have been restricted, to say the least.

The next week when she came in, she said, 'I don't know if the Time Line Therapy completely worked.'

'Really? Why is that?' I asked.

'Well, I was without anxiety for most of the week,' she said, 'but then one day I was driving along a certain road in a certain part of town, and when I got to a certain point I remembered something from when I was a child that had taken place there, but I had never remembered it till then. When I did I felt the terror and panic again.'

'Okay,' I said. 'Why don't you tell me what happened in that event.'

'We were driving along that road, and I had done something bad. I don't remember what. But my parents stopped the car, put me out on the side of the road, and drove off without me. I was terrified.'

'Oh dear. What a horrible thing to do to a child. Did they come back and get you?'

'I don't know. I don't remember. I suppose they must have.'

'I imagine that when they put you out, you really were terrified: that fear of death.'

'Oh yes. I was panicked.'

'And when you remembered it this past week, how frightened were you then?'

She thought. 'Well, I remembered how frightened I felt when it happened.'

'Exactly,' I said. 'And telling about it now, how frightened were you?'

'Not at all.'

'So remembering it now, those feelings of fear and anxiety, they are gone now?'

'Yes,' she replied, musingly.

'Well then, I think it did work. This sometimes happens. After TLT, sometimes a repressed memory emerges. It carries with it the "signature" of the original emotion. But not nearly as strong, and then it releases it.'

The idea that the mind can do this seems unbelievable to many traditionally trained therapists. It did to me initially when I read about it. But experience with TLT leaves me convinced that when the time is right and the client is ready, it can bring great change quickly. The funny thing is, clients are very matter of fact about the changes after the fact. I have had opportunity to inquire of clients many years later if the changes we made with the TLT are still good. The typical response is, 'Of course. Why do you ask?'

There Is a Principle

Whether you choose to learn NLP and utilize it or not is up to you. It is easy to learn and apply. For those who doubt its efficacy, may I respectfully refer to a quote from William Fraley, often attributed to Herbert Spencer, 'There is a principle which is a bar against all information, which is proof against all arguments, and which cannot fail to keep a [person] in everlasting ignorance—that principle is contempt prior to investigation.' Let me urge you to investigate it. You might like it.

LEARNING TO RECOGNIZE EMOTIONS

Though not a part of NLP, Paul Ekman's training in micro-expressions,[8] and recognition of emotions, generally,[9] is another similar approach to detecting emotional and, hence, physiological states by visual observation of facial expressions.[10] This is important for us as clinicians in order to detect the subtle and obvious emotions of our clients to understand how our interventions are affecting them.

It is also important to help the clients themselves identify their own emotional states. Often clients are unable to put a label on what they are feeling. It is important to be able to accurately identify our feelings because those feelings are what let us know what our needs are and also motivate us to meet those needs. This is the starting point for using MMH to identify needs and evaluate how our clients are going about getting those needs met.

Those emotions that are rooted in our physiology are key to guiding our choices and our behaviour. The emotions we *feel* are often different from the ones we espouse. This is particularly important when clients feel secondary emotions, for example, of shame and guilt, for not feeling the primary emotion of grief at the death of an abusive parent. These emotions are generated by the unconscious mind based on our needs.

Dream Work

The unconscious mind is a treasure trove of information just waiting to be got at. It is regularly giving us messages about what is going on around us and inside us in relation to what has gone on in the past. Sometimes those messages are coded, abstract, not obvious at all. Sometimes they are quite direct. Dreams are a direct link to the unconscious: what Freud called 'the royal road to the unconscious mind.'[11] Indeed they are, and it is important to remember that the traffic is two-way. That is, the unconscious mind uses dreaming to give us information, experiences, or insights that we might not otherwise have available to our conscious mind. Our conscious mind then influences our unconscious mind by our reaction to the information in the dream. The emotional reaction to the emotional content of the dream is, in effect, the instruction that we give to the unconscious mind to guide future behaviour. Here is an example of how this works.

Using Dreams

When patients came into the treatment centre and began to withdraw from their drug of choice, typically they would dream of using their substance again. We labelled these 'using dreams.' I noticed that these dreams seemed to follow a pattern.

The first phase would be dreaming that they were using their substance accompanied by euphoria. Euphoric recall is a problem in treating addiction disorder as fantasies of using again can trigger clients into leaving treatment. It is the siren's song. They would often awake feeling disappointed and thinking, 'Damn, it was just a dream!' These were the patients who were at risk of leaving treatment AMA (against medical advice).

Typically, they would have one of three reactions. First was to acknowledge that they wanted to leave treatment and use, sometimes doing so and sometimes not. Second was to deny wanting to leave but do it anyway. Third was fear that it meant they were *going* to leave and use, even though they did not want to.

Their unconscious mind was asking the conscious mind about this programme that was used regularly but hadn't been used in a while. What did the executive function (the mahout) of the mind want the unconscious mind to do with this programme? The patient's emotional response then determined whether they left treatment or stayed. If they stayed in treatment in spite of the euphoric recall, then we went to the next phase.

In this phase, the patient dreamed that they were going to use again, remembered that they weren't supposed to, and then did it anyway. They would feel guilty as they knew they were letting down their counsellor/loved ones/employer/etc. When they awakened the typical reaction was, 'Thank God! It was just a dream. Whew!'

I reassured the patients that it did *not* mean that they were doomed to leave treatment against their will. I pointed out the progress they had made: instead of feeling regret that they couldn't go out and use, they were feeling guilt about their using *in the dream*. That meant that their unconscious mind was incorporating the message: using was no longer desirable.

In the third phase they dreamed of having the opportunity to use, but they were very clear that they did not *want* to use, and they didn't. This led to waking up with a sense of satisfaction. This indicated they were likely to be successful in their recovery, because now they were internally motivated to remain sober. Their response of feeling pleased that they didn't use in the dream reinforced the instruction to the unconscious mind that they no longer wanted to use.

This is direct communication between the conscious and unconscious minds. The conscious mind has communicated something to the unconscious mind about drug use and sobriety. The unconscious mind has responded by dreaming a scenario based on the instructions that it has. The conscious mind has responded with a clarification of the instructions, Either, 'Oh, no, I don't want to do that,' or, 'Yes, please, I would like to do that,' or somewhere in between. The unconscious mind then does its best to carry out that instruction and will communicate further with other, similar, dreams that gradually change with time and the dreamer's intention.

In the treatment centre, a lot is happening in a short period of time, so the dream progression I have described can happen pretty quickly. In the real world, it takes longer. Next is an example of a dream that has taken longer to actualize.

The Accountant and the Artist

Gregory was very cognitively organized: A6, with perhaps a touch of C3–4, a pattern that I often see. His information processing was mostly cognitive. However, he would have massive 'INAs' (Intrusions of Negative Affect) where he shouted at and verbally abused his partner. With others he was polite and mild. Gregory had come to see me because he had broken up with this partner of many years and he was distressed by it, but equally he could not understand why he was so abusive to her. He was fearful of getting back with her. He realized that even though his outbursts were often in response to things that she did that annoyed him because they did not make sense to him, his outbursts were not always justified, even in his own mind. And even when they were justified, they were excessive.

Clearly, he had excessive anger directed towards his *attachment figure*, in this case his partner, and I suspected that it was coming from repressed anger towards his *attachment figure*, his mother. There was plenty of supporting evidence in the AAI for this hypothesis. The anger towards his father in the past was evident in his AAI, but he had decided, cognitively, that he was wrong to feel that way. But there was no expressed anger towards mom, except on one occasion where it was also expressed towards his father; thus, it was towards 'parents' as a team. More came from the Time Line Therapy® process: a very strong statement of unresolved anger at his mother. It was so strong and self-protective that we were unable to get at it.

His conscious mind report was that he did not remember much of his childhood until around age 7, where his explicit memories began. He did have some memories from prior to 7, but they were mostly in the form of vignettes. He had no memories of his older sister but did have some for his older brother. They were 4 and 6 years older, respectively. They came from an upper middle-class family and his parents had a wide social circle with lots of entertaining.

Though he could remember no anger at his mother, he did say that they were never very close, but neither was she ever unkind. His perceptions of his father were often of how his father related to his mother. He at several places had a negative view of how his father treated his mother, saying that he had thought his father 'boorish' for the way he had treated her, but then he would immediately retract it by saying that he realized later when he got to know his father as an adult that he had been wrong about that. So, no negative feelings towards mother to recall, negative feelings towards father but then retracted in adulthood.

Gregory was very precise in our early sessions about how he wanted the sessions to proceed. They were 2-hour sessions and he wanted 40 minutes to tell about how his week had gone and process it a bit, 40 minutes for the AAI work, and 40 minutes for REBT.

Some might argue that a cognitive approach is unhelpful for someone who is already cognitive, but that would be incorrect. This is because, at the higher levels, for example A6, cognition is significantly distorted. Gregory was perfectionistic to the point that when anyone associated with him, for example partner, children, even co-workers, got something wrong, he took it very personally as if he was responsible and it was an affront to him. A typical scenario was when his partner had to go somewhere. She was chronically late. Even when it had no direct effect on Gregory, he would become outraged thinking of the effect that it would have on other people.

Gregory had two dreams on the same night. In the first, Gregory was supervising a young male accountant. The accountant was to compile some figures for him so that he could give Gregory the results. They hadn't been done yet and Gregory was getting impatient. There was information missing that the accountant needed in order to complete the task. Gregory wasn't sure if he could believe the young man or not.

In the second dream a female artist had made a sandpainting mandala. But this one was different: sections of it could be removed and taken away. People had taken away sections of this artwork. Gregory thought, 'No that is wrong. They should be brought back because the artwork is not complete without them.'

Gregory could make no sense of it and neither could I, initially. Then suddenly it occurred to me what the meaning of the dreams was. This was not a 'figuring it out' process. Rather, it was a moment of intuitive understanding. The dreams belonged together as one dream in two parts. The structure was analogous to the two parts of the mind. The first dream represents the cognitive mind, the left hemisphere of the brain where facts and figures and logical processes live. The task set for the cognitive mind, to figure out what had happened during childhood so that he could make it all 'add up,' could not be completed because certain critical information was missing. Gregory's doubt about the young accountant's truthfulness indicates his own self-doubt.

The second dream represents the emotional, intuitive mind, where feelings and gut instinct rule. The artist's creation represented an 'experience' that was composed of different elements which can be separated out and taken away. When that happens, the experience cannot be recreated in its entirety. In order to get the experience, the pieces must be brought back so that the gestalt of the experience is complete. Only then can the information be given to the cognitive mind so that it can all 'add up' and make sense experientially, in the same way that memories are 're-membered.' You need all the 'members' to make a complete memory.

This encapsulated Gregory's dilemma: he was trying to figure things out cognitively but the elements of experience necessary—the emotions— were missing. What it gave us was an experiential talisman to which we returned over and over again as we did the therapeutic work to get back the missing pieces of the artist's metaphorical work.

NOTES

1. Ramacharaka, Y. (2007). *Science of breath: A complete manual of the oriental breathing philosophy of physical, mental, psychic and spiritual development*. Book Tree.
2. Nestor, J. (2020). *Breath: The new science of a lost art*. Penguin.
3. Porges, S. W. (2009). The polyvagal theory: New insights into adaptive reactions of the autonomic nervous system. *Cleveland Clinic journal of medicine, 76*(Suppl 2), S86.
4. https://www.youtube.com/watch?v=k7WNCalPbBQ.
5. LeShan, L. (2017). *How to meditate: A guide to self discovery*. Little, Brown Spark.

6. Erickson, M. H. (2009). Naturalistic techniques of hypnosis. *American Journal of Clinical Hypnosis, 51*(4), 333–340.
7. Adlerian Psychology—Life Style Analysis, Dr Harold Mosak, University of Alabama at Birmingham, Birmingham, Alabama, 1991, 11.5 hours.
8. https://www.paulekman.com/resources/micro-expressions/.
9. Ekman, P. (1999). Basic emotions. *Handbook of cognition and emotion, 98*(45–60), 16.
10. https://www.paulekman.com/.
11. Freud, S. (1983). The interpretation of dreams. In *Literature and Psychoanalysis* (pp. 29–33). Columbia University Press.

CHAPTER 7

Reorganization

AAI Processing—The Core

ACT is a dynamic, recursive process. What the analysis of the AAI is telling us about the client's functioning is attenuated by what the client's functioning is telling us about the analysis of the AAI. The AAI is a picture taken in a given set of circumstances at a given time and must be interpreted as such. I am working through the AAI *with* the client and forming a partnership *with* the client in order to deal with their feelings and meet their needs. If my hypothesis is correct about the strategy being used, then we should be able to predict new outcomes based on treating it as such. It seems that it is equally important to use what is happening in real life to understand what is being related in the AAI. What the client is actually doing and bringing to therapy on a regular basis is just as important to understanding the AAI as the AAI is to understanding what the client is doing and bringing to therapy. Each needs to inform the other.

I generally elicit the client's opinion of how they think they are functioning and how they functioned in the past. Sometimes they get it right, and other times they may have it 180 out. Regardless, we discuss the possibilities and the behaviour that is taking place to give evidence for our speculations. We also discuss how this strategy plays out in real life, and the client can then evaluate their own life circumstances and behaviours to see how well the theory fits the facts.

C. Shults, *Attachment Centred Therapy*, Palgrave Texts in Counselling and Psychotherapy, https://doi.org/10.1007/978-3-031-60851-3_7

I emphasize as we begin working that a theory explains observed behaviour or outcomes. It needs to be able to predict with some degree of accuracy what outcomes will be achieved by a particular course of action. When it does so, that establishes credibility for the client, and it also reassures me, as the coder, because I am *never* certain that I have got it right. In fact, to be open to getting it wrong, and to look for evidence of where and what we might have wrong, is a good way to test the theory and to make progress as new learning occurs.

> *I learn more when I admit that I am wrong*
> *than I do when I prove that I am right!*

If our theory of what strategy is at play is not supported by the observed evidence, then we must go back to basics, plug in the new information, and re-assess. This means going back to the beginning of our thinking about it with our new understanding to see what we come up with.

What is going on in the client's life is much more complex than a written classification can provide. Just as the map is not the territory, neither is the AAI classification the experience of the client. The map is a useful way to describe the subjects of interest, just as a classification is a useful way to describe the experiences of the client. They allow us to form hypotheses and make predictions based on those.

Many clients report that doing the AAI is transformative. Because of the way that it is structured and the nature of the questions themselves, it causes them to think of their past, and particularly their childhood, in a different way. Each time an event is 'remembered,' the 'members' of that event—the visual, auditory, kinaesthetic, olfactory, auditory digital, and neuroceptive components—are subject to varying degrees of degradation, magnification, deletion, and other forms of transformation that can cause these memories to change over time. In this way, we do 'change the past.'

Memory is never exact. This allows us to re-process our memories and 'remember' them differently. In this way, we can change how we relate to the past. We also correct errors. For example, instead of, 'My father beat me because I was a disobedient child,' we reintegrate the information as, 'My father beat me because he thought that was the best way to raise a child, based on his own abusive upbringing.' That is what Attachment Centred Therapy is about: changing the past so that we can have a better future.

RECONSTRUCTING HISTORY

Being able to give a coherent narrative of one's life is perhaps the most important indicator of mental and emotional health.[1] That was the most striking piece of information that I took from my training in counselling. I think that it struck me so strongly because it was the only one that I would not have included myself. 'How,' I thought, 'could simply giving a coherent narrative of one's life history be an *indicator* of one's mental and emotional health?'

At the time I was mystified, but now I know. Attachment Theory, and particularly the Dynamic Maturational Model of Attachment, explains why: because we base our actions in the here and now and our plans for the future on what has happened in the past. If our history, our internal record of the past, is incoherent and distorted, then that is going to impair our here and now functioning and our planning for the future. Some might even say that it would dictate it. The coherent narrative is a defining feature of Attachment Narrative Therapy (ANT) as well.

When we look at it that way, we realize that we are prisoners of the past. That theme has been developed over and over again. Alice Miller's book, *Prisoners of Childhood: The Drama of the Gifted Child*,[2] was written by her when she was a Freudian or Neo-Freudian psychoanalyst. The book is really a book about attachment and how it influences us throughout our lives and how psychotherapy can enable us to get free. Even more interestingly, when I re-read her book, the new edition had an introduction in which she wrote that having written the book, she had decided to eschew psychoanalysis. Why? Because it was part of the problem, she had concluded. Why was it part of the problem? In essence, the Freudian 'psychoanalyst/patient' relationship essentially replicated the stern, non-communicative authoritarian attachment relationships that had created the problems in the first place. In other words, it would actually help to perpetuate rather than heal the problems. At the time, I thought that she might be too harsh regarding her erstwhile therapeutic discipline. Since that time, I have had the opportunity to be associated with practitioners and recipients of psychoanalysis, and based on those experiences, I am sad to say that it seems to me that she is right.

IDENTIFYING DISCOURSE MARKERS

Just as discourse markers are the key to unlocking the AAI, they are also the key to reorganization. They give us both the means to understand how the client is processing information and also a method for correcting them. Let's start with a simple example of how this works.

Roger, in answering the questions on the AAI, often omits personal pronouns. He might say, 'Born in the U.K., moved around a lot. Had a brother but he died.' If this was all the information that we had available to us on which to make an assessment, we could surmise that Roger is using an A strategy, perhaps A6. The first and most distinct discourse marker is the failure to use the personal pronouns 'I' and 'we.' This is 'distancing.' Since that is an indicator of the A strategy, if Roger can start including those personal pronouns in his discourse, has he become more like a B3? And the answer is: Yes! He has become more like a B3. If Roger can learn to use information processing that is consistently B3, does that mean that he has changed his attachment strategy from A6 to B3? Again, yes, I think so. A more challenging aspect will be the lack of emotion and detail in relating the death of his brother. This is likely going to be UL, unresolved loss, or UT, unresolved trauma, depending on the circumstances of the death.

Now, I think I know what some of you might be thinking: isn't that artificial? Yes and no. In order to do that consistently and economically, Roger is going to have to practise doing those things until they become instinctive. To do that, he must become conscious of what he is doing that distorts information. He must learn what to do instead, and he must be mindful of that process so that he remembers to do it. Over time, with enough practice, new neural pathways will be created for processing information. (See *In Search of Memory* by Eric Kandel,[3] and *Molecules of Emotion* by Candace Pert,[4] both Noble Prize winners.) Those new ways of processing are going to lead to new outcomes. This is where knowledge of NLP, and particularly Ericksonian language use, can facilitate the process of reprogramming the mind.

Roger is going to be passing through the latter two of the four stages of learning: conscious competence, where he has to think about his information processing, eventually reaching unconscious competence. He has already passed through the first two stages: unconscious incompetence, where we don't know what we don't know; and conscious incompetence, where we know what it is that we don't know. For example, 'I know there must be a better way to go down the stairs, but I can't stop bumping long enough to figure it out!'

It is in conscious competence where we have to think about what we are doing. Someone in our training group came up with the clever slogan: Be Patient with Me, I'm an Earned B3! Meaning that I can get to the B3 position (or at least, head in that direction), but it takes me a bit of thinking about it to do it.

The final stage of unconscious competence I first recognized when a client told me of sitting on the beach and a couple came by, said hello, and began chatting with him. He answered and they had a nice conversation about the pleasure of being on the beach. He said that he would have never done anything like that previously and that he didn't consciously think about it. He just did it. It was only afterwards that he reflected on it and realized the difference in his behaviour. Previously, from his A5–6/C5–6 strategy, he would have given a minimal reply as a brush-off. Instead, he was surprised to realize upon reflection that he had eagerly engaged in the conversation and had quite enjoyed it. He was emotionally engaged. I have had many such reports from clients who had similar experiences.

It takes time and effort, but when it is done the effects are lasting and pervasive. So whatever amount it may cost in time, effort, and money, it will pay dividends for the rest of one's life.

These discourse markers, and the patterns that they form in the transcript, identify the attachment strategy that the person is using. If we look only at the transcript in order to determine the attachment strategy that the person is using, then we may be going astray. Context is vital: you can't understand the behaviour unless you understand the context in which it is used.

Dallos and Vetere discuss this in their book, *Systemic Therapy and Attachment Narratives*.[5] They are systemic therapists, and they start with the family system and apply attachment concepts and their own Attachment Narrative Therapy (ANT) in a wide variety of settings. I think of their approach as starting from the outside and working in to the individual, whereas my approach, Attachment Centred Therapy (ACT), starts from the individual perspective and then understands the individual from the perspective of the system—usually the family—in which they operate.

The other aspect that ACT has in common with ANT is the narrative aspect. The central proposition of ACT is that creating a more coherent narrative of one's life experience creates a healthier, more functional individual. I help clients to change their narrative from one that gives rise to the A or C strategies into one that gives rise to the B strategies. It is typical, when I am working through the transcript with the client, that they will often spontaneously utter statements that are sometimes word for word with what they have stated in the interview. For example, if I am reading a paragraph and read a sentence or two and then pause, they may spontaneously carry on with the very next sentence. Sometimes word for word, but when not entirely word for word, the narrative typically closely paraphrases what they said in the interview. This can go on not just for sentences but for whole paragraphs. Often, as I go through this process with clients, when we get towards the end of the transcript where the integrative questions are found, the client will spontaneously say, 'Oh, but I wouldn't answer that question that way today. I would answer it totally differently.' They will then typically go on to give me the new answer that does the things that we would like it to do: they are able to reflect on why their parents and others did what they did, how they may have contributed to the problem or failed to be protective of themselves or others, how they would respond differently today and project a new outcome for themselves into the future. This occurs spontaneously, without rehearsal or assistance on my part. This is another indicator that their unconscious mind information processing has been effectively reprogrammed.

You can see an example of this if you look back to Rehan's Lover, and his answer to the question, 'So, if you were upset emotionally what would you do?' Then compare it to the answer he gave when I asked for this book. His new answer was coherent, sympathetic to mom's motivations and her lack of ability to meet his needs, and the more subtle aspect of shaming him in the name of helping him through prayer.

ACT presumes that the therapist has established rapport, the essence of which is to relate to the client as one human being to another, not as 'the expert' who regards the client from on high. Rather, we are equals, first and foremost. Some clients may wish to defer to the therapist as the authority figure. Andrea is such a client. Others may wish to seem superior. In that case, it is important for the therapist to allow that positioning without assuming the role that the client has established for them. Rather, you, as therapist (or parent, partner, or whatever) need to maintain your own centre, your own position. Don't fall for the trap of being either superior or inferior.[6]

The approach I recommend is to allow the client whatever illusion they need to put onto you, while gently affirming that you are yourself, not who they think you are. Point out, when appropriate, that this is a projection of their own perception onto you, and that while you are willing to allow them to be where they are with it, you're not going to buy into it. Maintain your authenticity.

Either way, this gives you 'grist for the mill.' It is a vital part of the client's strategy: how they related to the interviewer (this may be yourself) at the time and how they are relating to you as their therapist now. It is information that you can incorporate into your treatment plan. When I say 'treatment plan,' this may or may not be a written document. There are settings where such a written formulation is appropriate and some where it is required. These were a staple in my first counselling role in the addiction treatment centre. If you haven't had experience with formulating treatment plans, I recommend you give it a try for your own edification.

For my purpose, it is the plan that I have in my mind, and so it, too, is fluid and dynamic. Lest it become untethered from reality, it is important to have anchor points or what I refer to as 'firm ground in the swamp.' It gives us a firm foundation from which to proceed. I hope I demonstrate what I mean by this in some of the case studies.

The maxim of manner, which means proceeding in a collaborative and cooperative manner, is meant to replicate the mother/child dyad where the child is dependent on the mother for guidance and getting needs met, and the mother is dependent on the child for emotional cues as to what is needed and for a response to what is offered. Of course, the therapist/client dyad has advantages that the mother/child dyad doesn't have. An articulated language is the first advantage so that we can use words to represent reality and to create imaginary realms where change can be explored. Remember, 'Words are more than mere concepts, they are the tools that we use to grasp and grapple with reality.'

That is why, after birth itself and the first step taken, the first word spoken is such a major milestone in a child's development. It is the grasp of the basic concept that words can be used to describe and designate concepts that are grasped by the first word! This is not to discount the non-verbal communication that conveys much more information. The language we use reflects the internal information processing that creates it.

As I read through the transcript, I point out each discourse marker or 'construct'—such as manner—when we get to it. I explain what it means generally in the overall scheme of the DMM and in my experience, and then if I have an idea of what it means in this particular context, I explain that as well. I then invite the client to comment on what they think about it, especially in view of the possible interpretation that I have given it. If I have one, that is. Sometimes I am simply baffled and ask the client for clarification. They may be able to provide enlightenment, or they may be baffled as well. In the latter case, I 'flag' the discourse marker so that we can return to it for further clarification once we have more information.

The process will go slowly at first, as there are lots to learn about. I encourage patience, with the assurance that it will gain momentum as we go and as they learn about the particular discourse markers and patterns that apply to them. I also make clear to them that this is collaborative, so what I am offering is my opinion of what I think I am finding. I encourage the client to form their own opinion of whether they agree, disagree, or just don't know yet.

ACEs: Adverse Childhood Experiences

This step-by-step approach allows the client to begin to explore which strategy they have used at various times in their lives. Attachment strategies will sometimes change as conditions alter and experiences influence interpretation of events. Going away to boarding school is a time of change for some, as are death, divorce, illness, psychosis, and other 'Adverse Childhood Events,' or ACEs. With proper support and resolution of negative feelings, ACEs don't doom one to attachment insecurity.

Some ACEs are going to require the client to shift strategy. For example, I had a client who started off with likely a B strategy. When her mother had a psychotic break when she was around 3, she shifted to an A strategy. The child had to assume a caregiving role for her mother. At the same time, and especially after the divorce that the psychosis precipitated, she had to accommodate herself to a rather inattentive father, meaning a C strategy was useful to get his attention. This then set her up for a marriage where she fell into a C strategy with her C4/A4 husband, who also had to organize around parents with differing strategies, all the while trying to maintain her A strategy in the rest of her life. I am happy to say that, last I heard, this couple is now doing well as they reorganize towards attachment security.

Many clients, as a result of experiences such as these, will have mixed strategies. They may alternate between A6, Compulsive Self-reliance, and C4, Feigned Helpless, for example. I find that mix often. The A4 Compulsive Compliance/Performance alternating with C4 is also typical, as is the A5/6 Compulsive Promiscuity and Self-reliance with the C5/6 Punitive/Seductive. The latter is a volatile mix that I encounter often when working with sexual addiction and compulsivity.

I want to reiterate that I believe the most significant ACE is simply not getting one's emotional needs met and not learning how to deal with one's feelings. Because this ACE of neglect occurs so early—from birth onwards, usually—it is deeply buried outside of conscious memory and that explains why clients have difficulty understanding and correcting their problems simply by talking about them. This trauma that—remember—caused many children to die from the lack of an attachment figure determines which strategy is going to be used and is going to provide the foundation for subsequent evolution of the strategy. Typically the A strategy is adapted in such situations.

We can always go through the transcript again and often do. Sometimes we will go back to earlier parts before we have finished the entire transcript. We go back and forth as needed and useful. As we learn more about the process, it imparts new meaning to earlier sections. Even with clients with whom I have been working for years, the AAI remains relevant, and we will refer to it when it seems beneficial.

Even when death does not occur to abandoned children, more subtle losses come from insecure attachment itself. NLP hypothesizes that we have an internal model for optimum functioning. We can identify certain manifestations of this that are undeniable. We know when we are hungry, thirsty, and tired. Our nurtural needs are not as certainly existential requirements but can result in death when they are not met. But what is the condition when we don't have our nurturing needs met but we don't die? We protest, then we become discouraged, and if we don't die, we adapt. This creates a legacy of shame, of worth-less-than-ness. This is loss.

As we mature, we are forced to compromise and accept less than our fair share of our needs being met. Just as a child denied proper nutrition is stunted in physical growth, so a child denied proper emotional nurturing is stunted in emotional growth. Coming to terms with that realization imparts an awareness of loss, and loss means grief. Let's consider each phase.

Dealing with Loss and Grief

People with insecure attachment are in a more or less constant state of unresolved grief that manifests in the various stages of grief that we are about to explore. That is the motivation for pursuing behaviours that relieve their suffering, if only temporarily and in spite of the behaviour making their situation worse. They are escaping from the fear of death. 9/11 gave us a graphic illustration of this phenomenon, collapsed into minutes rather than a lifetime.

There are obvious losses that the client was not able to grieve properly. Those are typically easy to recognize and plenty has been written about them elsewhere. The hidden loss, the one that, in my opinion, causes the most trouble, is the loss of secure attachment. I think that I have made that case sufficiently. In working with clients, the key is to be able to recognize when the client is entering the grieving phases. Clients will often deny that their attachment experiences have had an adverse effect on them. A+ clients will often insist that they had a perfectly good childhood when it is painfully evident from their AAI that they did not. For example, the client who relates that he was 'told off' by a parent for not wanting to do what her grandparents wanted to do. His wrap-up was that he was just being 'bratty.'

As clients progress towards a more balanced way of processing information and less distortion of the emotional and factual information, they will be able to look back on their past from a new height, shall we say, and perceive the losses that they suffered differently. And this realization will bring a recognition of loss, hence the need to grieve.

THE GRIEVING PROCESS

First described by Elizabeth Kubler-Ross in her book, *On Death and Dying*, her delineation of the grieving process I find essential in understanding where clients are in dealing with their losses. Not only that, the process of recovery, or reorganization, creates an awareness of loss. Whereas someone may have been doing a good job of denying any adverse impact from their childhood, going through the process of ACT is going to strip away the denial, allow the anger to emerge which can either (a) be turned inward into a form of non-curative depression (this could be the source of the Dp, or depression modifier? Being stuck in unresolved grief? And see the spin cycle further on). Expressed, the anger feeds naturally into blaming and bargaining. This *resists* going further into the next level of suffering of sadness and depression. This is the state of realizing the losses that your previous strategies and tactics have kept at bay. This is where the losses may be realized for the first time. If therapists and their clients don't realize this is going on, this effect may lead to further loss. The client may lose hope and leave therapy. The therapist may lose hope and wonder how they can endure their clients' pain and loss and hopelessness. But don't lose hope. This can be 'the dark night of the soul' that will lead to resolution and acceptance.

Denial

The grieving process starts with denial. This is manifest on the A+ side as false positive affect and on the C+ side in ignoring facts that are contrary to feelings. Denial comes in many ways. Be prepared for one layer of denial to be broken through, and a round of grieving processed and acceptance to be achieved, only to discover another layer of denial revealed that will set off a new round of grieving. Don't be discouraged. Even though you may be in the same phase, it will be at a deeper level. If your client is discouraged, point out the progress that they have made, and how the new round of grieving is based on a deeper understanding.

Anger

Anger is always about wanting something to change. In the case of insecure attachment, the ship has already sailed in terms of getting the nurturing that one needs. It actually *is* too late to have a happy childhood. However, it is not too late to resolve the losses, repair the damage, and be able to access the happy parts of childhood. When we are preoccupied with our negative feelings, whether indulging them or denying them, then we miss appreciating the good parts. When our anger is directed inwards towards ourselves, it becomes depression, self-hatred, or some other destructive emotion. Anger re-experienced is resentment. Resentment is toxic to our spirit. The best thing to do with anger from the past is to use it to motivate you changing yourself in the here and now.

Blaming and Bargaining

In this phase, we seek to hold someone accountable for the wrong. If this phase can help to bring about change, then use it. But most of the time, bargaining and blaming with attachment trauma is futile. Clients try to strike a compromise: If I do this (be a better son or daughter, try harder, etc.), then will you do that (be a better parent, more caring, etc.)? Many clients wish that their parents could be different than they are. They revisit the wrongs from the past in the hope of vindication. Or they blame themselves hoping that one day they will become 'good enough.'

The Spin Cycle

The spin cycle is when clients go round from denial, to anger, to bargaining and blaming, but instead of suffering the sadness and depression of the next level, they cycle back to denial and start the process all over again. They deny that their parents did the best they could and that they are powerless to change things. Be patient and persistent in challenging this.

Suffering of Sadness and Depression

I have added the term 'suffering,' meaning 'to allow,' to this phase. This phase must be 'allowed.' That is, it is an act of will to avoid the spin cycle and to avoid the use of some anaesthetic to avoid the suffering. The depression of this phase is different from anger turned inwards. This is the 'down,' 'blue,' or 'sad' depression. This suffering leads us to the next phase.

Acceptance

Acceptance means we have learned from the past and are ready to go into the future with new learnings, and a new awareness, that make it possible for us to have a happier, more fulfilling life. It means that we have reorganized ourselves in a more balanced way, becoming more secure.

Notes

1. Baerger, D. R., & McAdams, D. P. (1999). Life story coherence and its relation to psychological well-being. *Narrative inquiry, 9*(1), 69–96.
2. Miller, A., & Ward, R. T. (1981). *Prisoners of childhood: The drama of the gifted child and the search for the true self.* Basic Books.
3. Kandel, E. R. (2007). *In search of memory: The emergence of a new science of mind.* WW Norton & Company.
4. Pert, C. B. (1997). *Molecules of emotion: Why you feel the way you feel.* Simon and Schuster.
5. Dallos, R., & Vetere, A. (2021). *Systemic therapy and attachment narratives: Applications in a range of clinical settings.* Routledge.
6. Adler, A. (2014). Individual psychology. In *An introduction to theories of personality* (pp. 83–105). Psychology Press.

CHAPTER 8

Techniques for Working with Couples and Families

The primary difficulty in working with couples is each blaming the other. Sometimes, they fall into the pattern where one is top dog and the other is underdog. Top dog berates underdog and underdog tucks tail and cowers. Others go through cycles of being limerent with one another, then breaking up after the relationship has been consummated, and by that I mean become stable, living together, and so on. The new wears off and so does the thrill. And for those who confuse limerence with love, they begin to think that the love has gone. Spoiler alert, it wasn't there in the first place. It was love's illusion. They really don't know love at all. That is, they have some of the same neurological pathways involved, but not the 'willing to take a risk for the spiritual growth of self or other' variety.

Of course, each can see the other's difficulties quite clearly. If we look back at the grief process in the previous chapter, I will suggest that what many couples experience is the dis-illusion of their marital (partnership) experience and the first three phases, the spin cycle. Their struggle at the blaming and bargaining phase propels them back into denial: denial that it can ever get better; denial that either or both of them could make things better by focusing on the things *they* can change, *a la* the serenity prayer:

© The Author(s), under exclusive license to Springer Nature Switzerland AG 2024
C. Shults, *Attachment Centred Therapy*, Palgrave Texts in Counselling and Psychotherapy,
https://doi.org/10.1007/978-3-031-60851-3_8

> *Grant me the serenity*
> *To accept the things I cannot change*
> *Courage to change the things I can*
> *And wisdom to know the difference.*
> *Reinhold Niebuhr*

And the one thing we can change is ourselves, except … This is where attachment comes in.

We resist change out of fear. Because for an infant or young child, maintaining the caregivers protection is pre-programmed as an existential task. The risk of rejection and abandonment carries a deep sense of dread. Our responses to the environment are based on information from the past. It goes through our perceptual filters, our belief system, and comes out as a DR (dispositional representation) complete with slogans and emotions designed to whip up the mob of emotions buried in your brain. Hence, the need for reprogramming: for communication and cooperation. When couples begin to see one another as the enemy they divide into warring camps. Neither trusts the other.

This can propel the couple into the A versus C death spiral for the relationship. The person using the C strategy has a complaint about an issue. They express it as a criticism of the other person, or, expressing it inexactly, the other person using the A strategy hears it that way. That is why it is so important to use the 'What I heard you say is' part of the couple's communication technique, or, conversely, 'Hold on, what did you just hear me say?'

When the A strategists hear the complaint as a criticism, then they are likely to respond defensively. They may pull away physically, emotionally, or both. Often they go into the 'flop' mode and don't respond at all, effectively 'playing dead.' The C then escalates their demands, perhaps going into character assassination, the A withdraws even more, and the cycle for the relationship goes downward in the death spiral.

Sometimes what keeps the couple from splitting up is having a child. The child may become the focus of their unresolved negative feelings. This child then becomes the 'identified patient.' Sure enough, they live down to their parents' expectations and dutifully play out the role they have been assigned. Or, if they rebel, that becomes further evidence that they are the problem. The child has become the symptom carrier for a dysfunctional relationship.

This becomes the scapegoat child. Paradoxically, I have had several clients, individually and in the family context, who, by becoming the scapegoat, actually became more successful and responsible than any of their siblings. These were dysfunctional families and in context to be the black sheep was a good thing. An older child had taken the 'hero' position, whose accomplishments proved that the family was alright. This means the second child is relegated to the scapegoat role, so while the hero can do no wrong, the scapegoat can do no right. There may be a lost child, exemplified by wondering, 'Where's Chris? I haven't seen him all weekend?' 'Oh,' my sister replied, 'he's in his room playing dungeons and dragons.' The role of family hero was taken by his oldest sister, and the middle sister was the scapegoat.

In one case, the client was one of non-identical twins. His mother was quite obviously fond of and favouring of the other, and putting down and criticizing my client. But in adulthood, the favoured twin had become a ne'er-do-well, while my client had become a rather heroic figure in real life, with accomplishments that won him great respect and admiration.

In other cases, the child becomes triangulated into the couple's difficulties, becoming an ally for one against the other. Or, as in the case of Rehan, the child plays a peacekeeping role. In neither case is this going to be optimal for meeting the child's needs.

The key to these situations is to help the couple to become more resourceful in dealing with their own issues. This means, if possible, to get the couple to do their individual work using the AAI. The focus becomes how what we are finding in the AAI is reflecting the issues in the couple's relationship. However, not all couples are keen to do that, especially when it means giving up on the myth of the misbehaving child.

GOTTMAN AND THE SEVEN PRINCIPLES FOR MAKING MARRIAGE WORK

When I work with couples, typically I begin with the Gottman inventory, which is a series of questionnaires about their experiences interacting with one another. These can be found in his book, *The Seven Principles for Making Marriage Work*.[1] His concept is to build a 'sound marital house' using the tools given in his book. I have combined these inventories into a workbook, together with the Locke-Wallace Marital Adjustment Scale, that I send to clients to complete.

When I get the inventories back from the clients, I score them, and then I create a profile in an Excel spreadsheet where I can display the scores for each questionnaire, colour coded so the safe, marginal, and critical categories can be seen easily. I go over it with the couple, starting with the most critical. As Dr. Gottman emphasized, by focusing on the critical scales, the most progress can be made the quickest. By creating the profile, it is easy to see, visually, how they compare and where to start work to get the most results the quickest.

The Four Horsemen

Usually 'The Four Horsemen' are the most critical. The Four Horsemen are criticism, defensiveness, contempt, and stone walling. Although these can occur in different orders, I will deal with them here in the order given as that is the one you are most likely to encounter.

It is important to understand the difference between criticism and a complaint. We don't want to shut down complaints. If you have a complaint, it is important to voice it and be heard. Complaints are often accompanied by anger, perhaps in a lesser form such as irritation or annoyance. It is vital to express anger in relationship in the appropriate way. When we don't, the anger can build up into resentment, and resentment is toxic.

A complaint might be, 'You didn't put the bins out and now we will be overloaded with trash. I'm really annoyed.' A criticism about the same event might be, 'Why didn't you put the bins out? You never do what you're supposed to. Why can't you be more responsible?' The first focuses on a specific issue and identifies a problem with behaviour. It induces guilt, and the listener can rectify the situation by changing the behaviour. The second starts with the specific issue but in an inquisitorial manner. It then seamlessly segues into character assassination. It induces shame because there is little the listener can do to rehabilitate their character.

Defensiveness naturally follows character assassination. The listener can agree with the complaint and take corrective action. The criticism is pervasive and overly broad. The listener can remember many times when they *did* do what they were supposed to, and so they may defend by protesting the validity of the criticism. They also may try to mount a counter-attack by pointing out all the times when they thought the speaker was irresponsible.

When the first speaker, who had a legitimate complaint, perceives the listener as being defensive to the criticism, they respond with contempt.

'There you go again,' said with a roll of the eyes. In the face of the speaker's withering contempt and character assassination, the listener chooses to disengage completely, having been down this path so many times before and knowing that there is not going to be a good outcome.

Turning Toward, Away, or Against

Turning toward is a simple concept. When one partner makes a 'bid for affection,' wanting to speak, share some information, any overture that presents an opportunity for interaction, it is important that the other partner respond by, literally, turning toward them and engaging. We can't always do that. For couples to be happy in relationships, they need to do this at the least a majority of the time. And 80% of the time is a good target. Anything less than 60% is asking for trouble.

When the partner responds by turning away, this is going to harm the relationship. It takes time for this to erode the relationship to the point of dissolution. Short of 20 years based on Dr. Gottman's studies. Just the right amount of time to get married, have children, and then rock along, till they are mostly grown, to divorce. A pattern that we see a lot.

Turning against is even worse. A turning against response would be, 'Don't bother me now. Can't you see I'm watching the game?' Or, 'Well I don't blame your boss. If it's as hard for him to get you to help out as it is for me, it's no wonder he chewed you out.' These relationships only last 6–8 years according to Gottman, and likely are what give rise to the 'seven year itch' phenomenon.

Gottman's work is predicated on being able to create healthy relationships by following his suggestions. The longest questionnaire is the Shared Meanings and Dreams. These questions are about things that you can do to make the relationship stronger. In this regard it matches the 'Goals and Values' level of my Relationship Actualization model.

NOTARIUS AND MARKMAN AND THE RELATIONSHIP BANK ACCOUNT

Clifford Notarius and Howard Markman were graduate students of John Gottman so they draw on the same body of research. They authored a book together,[2] and then Notarius and Markman published their own book, *We Can Work It Out*.[3] In their book, they give brief versions of REBT, though they don't call it that. They also give instructions for the couples communication exercise. Their concept is of a relationship 'bank account.' Successful interactions (turning toward) make deposits while unsuccessful interactions (turning away or against) make withdrawals.

I debated whether to address the next point or not. Dr. Gottman disavows this 'active listening' approach. He said so in the training that I attended. He explained that his graduate student observers had finally confessed to him that the 'active listening' approach on which *A Couple's Guide to Communication*, and which Dr. Gottman had been advising for years, was rarely if ever used by his 'Master Couples' that they were observing in the marriage lab. Based on this he concluded that the active listening approach was useless.

I was puzzled. I had learned the active listening approach in my early days in the addiction treatment centre and later from Notarius and Markman's book, *We Can Work It Out*. I preached it to my clients. But Dr. Gottman's commentary made me think. Did I actually practise it? I resolved that I would attend to my own communications with my clients to see when, if at all, *I* used active listening. After a couple of weeks, I was beginning to doubt its efficacy, as I had not used it once, so far as I could tell. I was about to conclude, as Dr. Gottman had, that it really was not useful and to quit encouraging my clients to use it. And then it hit me.

It was the shock of recognition that I felt when I realized what I had just said: hold on, what did you just hear me say? I said this in response to a client who had, evidently based on their response, misunderstood what I had just said. Sure enough, they had misunderstood what I was meaning to communicate. The next words out of my mouth were also automatic, but I was aware when I said them. 'I'm sorry, I didn't make my meaning clear. Let me say it again.' This latter response implicitly puts the onus on me, the speaker, to make myself clear, which I proceeded to do in the session and we carried on productively. (Systemic Family Therapy and Attachment Narrative Therapy call this meta-communication.[4])

This was a revelation. I was using the active listening technique, and it was on automatic. Then I reevaluated what I had heard Dr. Gottman say. Notice, I just used it in the previous sentence. 'What I heard you say' is very different from 'What you said.' I had heard, 'My graduate students told me that the master couples we observe in the marriage lab don't use active listening often, if at all. I therefore conclude that it is useless and no longer advocate it.'

The above experience with my client when I used it suggested an appropriate analogy to me. 'What I heard you say is …' or its corollary,

'What did you hear me say?' is like rolling a kayak: (1) You only need to do it when you are upside down (when you or your partner haven't understood what was said or you want to be sure it was heard accurately). (2) You need to practise it enough so that you can do it automatically when needed. (3) Once you get that good at using it, you will be good enough (in your communication—or your kayaking!) that you rarely if ever need to use it.

Dr. Gottman's conclusion is illogical. It's as if someone was watching an Olympic whitewater kayaking competition and, noticing that none of the competitors used a roll, concluded that learning to roll a kayak wasn't necessary for Olympic competition.

In the same way, for two weeks of therapy sessions I had not used my active listening skills overtly. But then, when they were needed—when my client and I were metaphorically upside down in the water—I hit the metaphorical roll automatically and effectively by saying, 'Hold on, what did you just hear me say?'

With couples, I imagine that the Master Couples had grown up using their active listening skills rather than learning them as they got older. I also imagine that these Master Couples were probably in the secure categories of attachment, especially in their relationships. And keep in mind, these Master Couples were in the marriage lab to be observed. They weren't there to learn from the researchers but the other way round.

So, reading and understanding the basics of this active listening technique will be virtually useless unless you do these three things: practise, practise, and practise.

I Feel … When … Because …

This is a simple formula that accomplishes certain very important things. First, it starts with taking ownership of one's subjective impression. That is, a feeling. Feelings are one word. 'I feel like running away,' isn't a feeling. It is an expression of an action you are contemplating taking as a response to a feeling. 'I feel afraid,' is the likely feeling motivating this behaviour. We can easily reverse engineer the communication, 'I feel like running away,' and presume that the person feels fear. We are right often enough that this way of expressing feelings gets us by most of the time. Unfortunately, because we use these expressions as a sloppy way to express emotions, they can be easily misunderstood and the response may be counter to what we desire.

For example, the speaker might say, 'I feel like you aren't telling me the truth.' This is a problematic communication. 'You aren't telling me the truth' isn't a feeling, it's a statement of fact. 'I think you aren't telling me the truth' makes it a suspicion, an assessment, an assertion, and implicitly an accusation of lying.

The listener might respond with, 'Oh, now you're calling me a liar!' It's easy to see where this is headed!

That is when you need to use active listening. You don't need to ask, 'What did you hear me say.' They just told you what they heard. Don't respond with defensiveness: 'I DID NOT. I JUST CAN'T TRUST YOU.' Whoa!

Instead, try, 'I'm sorry. I didn't make myself clear. I am feeling anxious and suspicious. That's what I could have said.'

The listener still might hear it as an accusation. But at least the framework has shifted. Even better, if the first speaker can own, 'It's my issue. It reminds me of my previous partner who used to lie to me all the time—oh, I mean, quite often—in situations like this. So please try to understand that I feel insecure and suspicious based on past experience, and I really mean to be asking for your reassurance.' Whew. No wonder we engage in shortcuts like, 'I feel like you aren't telling me the truth.' Like I say, they are shorthand ways to speed communication and cooperation. But, and this is especially true in couples' communication: haste makes waste. Slow down and take your time. Instead of reacting angrily and trying to change things before you understand, be curious about why your partner, with whom you have chosen to spend your life, presumably, could be thinking, feeling, and saying whatever it is that you are angry, hurt, or ashamed about.

As with the REBT, in order to use active listening smoothly when you need it, you need to practise it when you don't need it. And remember, you can't learn to roll a kayak in the middle of a rapid, and you can't learn to use this method in the middle of a heated argument with your partner.

When you do get a response that doesn't make sense, it is useful to ask the other person, 'Hang on, what did you hear me say?' Couples often, and typically, in my experience, when they are coming for couple's therapy, are in the habit of misunderstanding one another. That is because we are often prepared for the worst and so we are already in the triple F of freeze, fight, or flight. In this state, which is activation of the sympathetic nervous system, we are primed to detect only threat. Oftentimes what the partner means as a peace offering, or a request for comfort, is taken as a threat instead. That's why it is important to clarify the meaning.

What I Heard You Say Is

This is the other half of the couple's communication exercise, 'What I heard you say is … Did I get that right?' This accomplishes several things at once.

Listening

First, it requires the listener to concentrate on what is being said. What often happens is that after the first few words are spoken, the person being addressed has gone off into their mind planning their rebuttal. Based on this 'preparing to defend' approach, the 'listener' often hasn't listened at all and gets the exact opposite of what the speaker is saying.

Understanding

The second thing that it does is to make sure that you have understood what is being communicated. In the following example, Bob hears Tanya saying that she doesn't want to be with him anymore, that they are not 'right for each other.'

> I mean we talked yesterday and, you know, Tanya was saying, 'You don't really understand me. You don't ask any questions. You don't know my dreams and aspirations,' you know? And I thought … it made me angry, and, in, you know … and this is progress: maybe three months ago I would have stewed on it, and then came out later, but actually I went, 'No, you are right.' And then, so my immediate reaction was, 'Then perhaps I am not right for you,' you know?

This illustrates two points about the A and C relationship dynamic. First, C's often express their desire for closeness as a criticism of their partner. Second, A's often hear this as 'You're not good enough, therefore, you are worthless.' They then respond to this request for closeness, which they interpret as criticism, defensively and withdraw or threaten withdrawal. This withdrawal is then threatening to the C+ and they respond by escalating their negative affect:

> Yeah. You know, she gets quite upset when I say, 'Well, perhaps I am not right for you.' And it's like, 'That's a threat. I don't want you to go.' I said, 'It's not a threat it's an observation.'
> **And she is right**.
> What? It is a threat?

Yeah.

Yeah?

Yeah. It is a threat. But, you are not meaning it as a threat. What you are reacting to is: it's as if what *she* said was a threat.

Yeah ...?

So, you are just countering her threat.

Yeah, okay ...

You don't see it that way because you interpret what she is saying as a threat.

Right. Okay.

But it's not. This is what I mean when I say, 'Install the "translator" in your mind that allows you to hear that, not as a threat, but as an invitation to come closer.'

Yeah. No. I can see that, and as I said, that is what she was trying to explain, but I did struggle with it a little bit. But I do understand it now, Charley. So, that's important that I understand it. That gives me a bit of clarity and also it lifts my mood a little bit in all honesty, Charley.

Just interacting with someone that you love, and who loves you, ought to be pleasurable. The trouble is, when you have experiences such as you had in childhood, you learn that, instead of being pleasurable, those interactions are painful. They are necessary because you have to do these things in order to get along in life, but it's not a source of comfort or pleasure for you *per se*, and that goes with the avoidant strategy, okay? (He nods) The avoidant strategy does not take pleasure in relationships, they take pleasure in pleasing other people that they are in relationship *with*, but instead of just hanging out and having fun, they put it in terms of 'Having To Do Something.'

Yeah.

And getting the money in is an excellent example of Having To Do Something. And it's complicated by other people's reactions. 'Well, you know, why aren't you happy? Why aren't you excited?' Well, you learn when you shut down the negative feelings, in this case the anger ...

Just run through it again though, just—those words again?

Well, you don't learn that it's essential to voice your displeasure when you feel it in order to keep the relationship healthy. Having those kind of conversations, Bob, is not an indicator that you are not right for one another. Hell no. It's an indicator that you're working together better and better going forward to get both your needs met and deal with your feelings effectively. What do you think of that idea?

Yeah, no that's good. Again, the conversation in the last 45 minutes, I can understand that because it's a level of clarity. If I had that conversation with Tanya previously, I would have just got up and walked out and gone, 'Fuck it, I'm gone. I don't need this shit.'

Yeah, exactly.
That tells me quite a lot. That tells me there is a level of maturity there, and also thinking, 'This is worth working at,' you know? Which is important.

If Bob could say, 'What I heard you say is,' it would be something like, 'I don't want you anymore. Go away.' Then Tanya could reply, 'No, that isn't what I meant at all. I'm saying that, when you don't ask me about my goals, even though I've asked you about yours, I think that you don't care about me.'

Sharing
The third thing this accomplishes is that the speaker 'feels heard.' That is short hand for, 'The speaker feels good/satisfied because they perceive that they have been heard and understood by the other person. This is the feeling of rapport.' Bob is feeling this in our session:

> That was a good conversation because it was on a different level. I don't know how to explain it. I felt that was a two way conversation. Does that sound stupid after all the times we've talked?
> **You and me?**
> Yeah. I just felt that conversation there was a proper two way conversation where I took in what you said and came back with what I thought.
> **You did. You are absolutely right. I see what you mean.**
> I heard what you said, thought about it, and came back, which is good …
> **Yes …**
> That's made, that has made me quite emotional that has … (voice trembling, eyes blinking)
> **Oh good. Enjoy that feeling.**

This is the first time that Bob has allowed himself to show and share these tender feelings of vulnerability in our sessions. Now, if he can just bring himself to do that with Tanya.

RELATIONSHIP ACTUALIZATION

Regardless of the particular techniques, the model that I use for couples is Relationship Actualization. In keeping with the spirit of Maslow, who studied how to make things better and to actualize our full potential, Relationship Actualization is intended to be a guide to a healthy, happy relationship.

Necessity was the mother of invention. Because I worked with so many clients who, in their compulsive sexuality and compulsive limerence had been in failed relationships in the past, they needed a guide for relationships in recovery—a relationship that would last and that could provide them with emotional satisfaction. There wasn't one, and I thought that we therapists needed to be able to answer a simple and straightforward question.

It seemed intuitively correct that the basis of an attachment relationship to another person was a spiritual attraction. And many of the clients that I worked with were participating in 12-step programmes, and part of the 12-step wisdom is that addiction is a spiritual illness. As such it requires a spiritual solution. I hope you understand my use of the term 'spirit' as being based on the spirit that enters our body with the first breath that we take and that leaves the body with the last breath we take. I have no desire to debate whether that 'spirit' is eternal, created by a supernatural being, a solipsistic result of reductionistic biochemical and electrical interactions in the brain, or whatever. For me it is not based on 'belief,' but rather on observation.

That gave me a starting point. As self-transcendence was at the top of the modified hierarchy, it occurred to me to simply turn the model upside down. I was pleasantly surprised to discover that the natural progression of the levels made sense to me as a developmental model for a relationship, hence, Relationship Actualization:

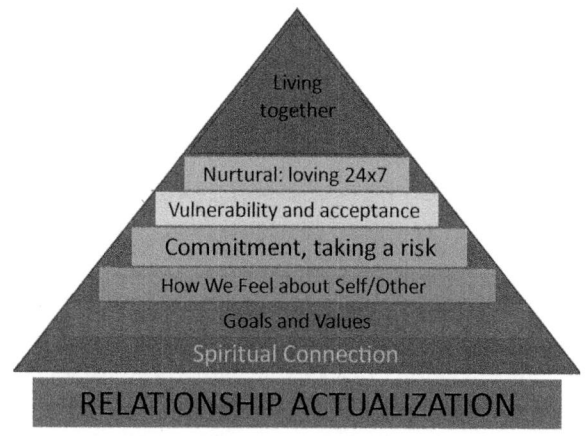

Spiritual Attraction

Beginning at the bottom, analogous to an individual's self-transcendence, is the couple's spiritual attraction. This is about being moved to abandon your own individual identity and become a part of something larger to which you give yourself. Just as physical needs, the bottom level of Maslow's Modified Hierarchy applies to everyone, so too, at the level of spiritual connection, we can relate to all beings on the planet. For that special person, however, we feel a special connection that attracts us to them and them to us, in addition to the physical attraction. It is somewhat ineffable, but I have had many clients recognize and describe that attraction in ways that were unique to them. This spiritual attraction grows over time and is the basis for lasting relationships. And, by the way, for the hopeless romantics who may be reading this, it is not to suggest that there is 'The One' that you simply must find. You make your partner into 'the one for you' by the relationship that you share.

Goals and Values

Once this attraction is experienced and both parties are agreeable, it is time to explore the next level that coincides with self-actualization/spiritual awakening. The essence of this level is to become the best that we can be, and in order to do that we must use our goals and values as a guide. Questions to ask are:

Are our goals and values compatible?
Can we support one another in actualizing our goals and values?
Will we be able to evolve and mature over time together?
Are we able to give ourselves shared meaning in life?
Can we take satisfaction from our partner's achievements?

If so, we are good to go. If no, then we need to look elsewhere. When your goals and values are not compatible, then you are asking for trouble in your relationship.

One client starting to date someone asked me if they were going too fast. She had been on a couple of dates and they had begun talking about their life goals. She wondered if they needed to get to know one another better first. I assured her that they *were* getting to know one another and that it was important to know if their goals and values were compatible before they got hooked. If there was incompatibility, best to discover it now.

Feelings About Self and Other

This coincides with the esteem level of need. The questions to ask here are:

> How do I feel about my partner when I am with them?
> How do I feel about myself when I am with my partner?
> How does my partner feel about me when they are with me?
> How does my partner feel about their self when they are with me?

These questions detect whether you have uncomfortable feelings, such as embarrassment, when you are with your partner. Whether you feel put down or shamed. Any uncomfortable feelings. Ideally, I suggest a mutual admiration society of two.

Unfortunately, sometimes getting close to someone that you really admire and desire can backfire through the Groucho effect: 'I wouldn't want to belong to any club that would have someone like me as a member!' This indicates that you need to work on your own self-esteem and self-worth issues. You are projecting your own sense of inadequacy onto your partner. 'If they want to be with me, there must be something wrong with them.' This is a hangover from the previous limerent feelings that told you, 'this is the one.' The one that is going to save you, to make you feel good about yourself, to prove your self-worth because, 'Look who (what, objectifying) I've pulled,' in a vain attempt to gain respect and admiration.

Unfortunately, some people, because it fits with what they have absorbed at the unconscious mind level, are 'comfortable' with being mistreated because it is what they know and what they think they deserve. For others, it is the other way round. They believe it is their duty to criticize and correct their partner. Obviously, these issues are only going to get worse as time goes on and are best to be avoided.

Commitment, Extending Yourself to Another

This is the level of love and belonging. If we have passed the tests at the first three levels, we are then ready to consider whether to make the commitment to ourselves and our partner that we are willing to take a risk, to extend ourselves, for the spiritual growth of both of us. It is this spiritual growth that sustains and deepens the relationship through time.

It is also about a commitment to do what is best for the relationship, even if it means a sacrifice of one's individual needs. This need not result in diminishment. To the contrary, it is about the spiritual growth that allows both of you to reach your full potential. That is why it is essential to successfully answer the questions for the three previous levels.

The questions for this level are:

> Are my partner and I willing to make a commitment to one another?
> Am I willing to take risks with and for my partner and our spiritual growth?
> Do we feel an attachment bond to one another?
> Can we treat one another with love, equality, and respect?

I like the suggestion from Notarius and Markman:[5] to treat your partner as pleasantly as you would a guest in your home.

Vulnerability and Acceptance

This is the level of safety and security. Here, we are willing to be truly known by our partner: our deepest fears, insecurities, and failings. It is also where we are called upon to accept our partner as they are, not try to change them. It's okay to ask for change, and of course, we will say how we feel about behaviours. But vulnerability and acceptance are the keys to feeling safe and secure in the relationship.

The first client I shared this with was puzzled. Because he was in the 12-step programmes, he had taken the words from the Big Book, about 'grasping and developing a manner of living that requires rigorous honesty,' to mean that he must tell any woman he was dating all the bad stuff he had ever done during his addiction on the first date! And he wondered why they ran away as fast as they could!

'No,' I explained. 'First, they need to get to know you. Yes, you did some pretty rotten things in your addiction, but that is not who you truly are. Let them get to know you in your recovery first, to feel your attraction to one another as human beings in the here and now, to evaluate your character via your goals and values, to experience how you treat them on a daily basis, and, if based on that information they have decided they want to go ahead with you, then do so. From a position of knowing who you really are in the here and now, and from having made a commitment for spiritual growth, they can properly evaluate any historical information that you need to give them, and vice versa.'

The questions here are:

> Am I willing to be vulnerable with my partner?
> Am I willing to be completely known by my partner?
> Am I willing to accept my partner as they are and not try to change them?
> Is my partner willing to accept me as I am and not try to change me?

The change part can be tricky. Of course, you are going to change and grow together. However, it needs to be up to each partner how they change. If you love one another, then why would you not want to please one another? So if your partner expresses annoyance or some other negative feeling, 'Please don't leave the toilet seat up!', 'Please remember to empty the dishwasher,' then it makes sense to change. However, the motivation needs to come from within, because you desire to please your partner. Not from without because she is nagging you!

Nurtural

Interestingly, this is the only level where I have used the same name in both hierarchies. I think that is because the nurturing need is the same, both going and coming back. This is where we touch, cuddle, smile, and say sweet things to one another. This means loving gestures, smiles, hugs, kisses, kind words, thoughtfulness, repair when things mess up, and so on. When you are able to do this with one another consistently, then you will be equipped to assist one another in raising children and you will have the capacity to nurture your children effectively too. The mechanisms are the same. Only now, adult sexuality has been added into the mix.

Some questions to ask at this level:

> Are my partner and I willing and able to be loving and caring of one another?
> Can we express our love with sex without shame, embarrassment, or repression?
> Can we express our love and caring without having sex?
> Can we work through our negative feelings effectively and get our needs met in a mutually supportive manner?

Living Together

This is the physical level. The realm of joint bank accounts, doing the chores, school runs, who's going to make the coffee, dinner, bed, and all the other details of daily living. It is the physical level of existence. Questions to ask here are:

Can we work together cooperatively to meet and manage the daily tasks of living?

Can we support one another when the demands of life are extreme?

Can we keep a proper perspective on the important things when life gives us setbacks?

Can we agree on what is important to us in living and can we be respectful of our differences?

A Useful Guide

Relationship Actualization is intended to be a guide to forming a relationship and moving through the different levels of the relationship as it forms. I also use it to help people evaluate where they are in the relationship and how they are doing at getting their needs met. Of course, a less than satisfactory evaluation could be due to something that their partner is doing, or it could be an unmet need based on the individual's difficulties. Trust is a good example. If one person is not feeling very safe in the relationship and is telling themselves they can't trust their partner, is that because the partner is doing something questionable, or is it because the person is suspicious and has difficulty trusting?

Here is an example of its use in a session. This is not about trust, but rather, spiritual growth:

[Session] **Okay Sue let's go for it.**
I really want to talk about my relationship with Larry. I have been thinking about that and I was wondering if it was possible that you could ask me questions about the relationship, because I am struggling to separate out the issues and I think being asked questions might help me.
Well, you are in luck. We will use Relationship Actualization. The first question is, do you feel a spiritual attraction with Larry?
That is a really hard question to answer, because I think I fell in love with Larry on the basis of a spiritual connection. There was lots of physical attraction as well, but the spiritual attraction was about the person that he was. Larry comes from a very working class family. Unskilled labour and a big family, with all your traditional ideas about racism, homophobia, you know? He had completely different ideas and ideals than his community. I saw him as somebody who was intuitively reflective and open, and him having had no experience educationally of learning any of those things, I was really attracted to that. So I think that was a real spiritual connection. I felt like his core sense of himself was exactly what I was looking for. There was another moment where he came to our house, and there was a bird stuck behind the

chimney, and [he rescued the bird]. That was like a real connection to think that he cared so much about something else's distress. So I think there was a really deep spiritual connection between us when we first started. Now I feel that there isn't so much of a spiritual connection between us. I feel like there is a real disconnect actually.

Okay, so something has happened to that. We will go onto the rest of these questions, that might give us a clue. Ideally that spiritual connection would grow over time.

Yeah.

Next is goals and values. Basically, what you want to get out of life and how you want to live your life. So, are your goals and values compatible is the first question?

(sighs) Probably not.

Oh?

I don't know how to answer that question. I suppose I have to identify what my goals are. My values are very much on this spiritual journey about getting to know me. Getting to know my place in the world. Being open to understanding new things. Being reflective, constantly learning. So that is part of my values. My goal is about providing more creative ways of being to connect to other humans in a way that kind of makes a difference to their life and mine.

Wow. Yeah.

I do feel that I should pay my clients, you know? Cause I learn stuff from them, and obviously, not just saying that in a kind of superficial way. There is something that happens in the dialogue between people that helps me.

Yes, absolutely.

I am genuinely curious. I am not asking questions because I know the answer. And I feel that that is my purpose in life—I really feel strongly that is my purpose and it's a purpose I have given myself. I don't feel like it's come from anywhere else. It's a purpose that I have given myself so that can be a kind of lifelong thing, really. It helps me feel not too overwhelmed by what is going on in the world cause it makes me feel like I can influence my part of the world, you know? And if there were more people who had open and reflective skills then what is going on in the world today wouldn't be happening.

Amen!

But I am not sure that matches with Larry's goals. Larry's goals are about— I don't even know whether he could articulate what his goals are, I think that his goals are about providing for his family, feeling like he does a good day's work, feeling that he is valued in the job that he does and that he is ethical. He would never skimp on his taxes. He is a socialist at heart. He believes in community and society and contributing. So his goals are more about providing for the family and contributing to society, and maybe making enough money to go on nice holidays and share nice times together. Those are his goals, so they are not completely different from mine. I think I would probably hold those goals as well in terms of providing for the family and society and that, so they are not too dissimilar. But also his goals are quite static. I mean at some point he will have to retire and *then* I'm concerned about what is going to happen then because he has no other real goals in life. [emphasis added]

Well, I really hear that he is a very honest person and very motivated by fairness, yeah?

Very motivated by fairness, very. Although sometimes it's his own version of fairness. Sometimes I see an unfairness where he doesn't see the unfairness, so you know, emotionally, often he is a nine year old boy. He takes things so personally.

Does he? Well back to spiritual growth: so that is one of the challenges of spiritual growth: to not take things personally.

Exactly. he takes everything personally. [She tells a story of the cat looking 'side-eye' at him] I think that is just a really good example of how Larry is constantly looking, is constantly suspicious of people. He is waiting for people to be critical of him so that he can defend himself. And that often includes me.

Well, that's something maybe that you would want to talk about? And if you haven't talked about your goals and values then maybe that would be a place to start?

With him?

Well, it's just a suggestion, you know?

I have already had that conversation with him and he said, 'I can't be you and I don't want the things that you want, I don't want to go on this spiritual journey that you have been on.' So he has already been fairly clear, really, about, his sense is, 'I've done enough.' He has benchmarks of people that he knows from his early childhood, that he has done better than them. He has moved out of the area that he lived in. He isn't racist, sexist, homophobic. He is thoughtful and considerate. He is a socialist. He feels that he has done enough to come further, and he is more emotionally intelligent, and all those things, so he has done enough. 'I'm done.'

How do you feel about that?

I feel like we are really stuck.

Okay, now. Can I be Mr REBT here and say that's not a feeling, that's what you are telling yourself? How does that *feel*?

I feel sad.

Sad, okay.

I feel really sad, yeah.

Mm
Really sad.
Okay. So basically you think the two of you are stuck and you feel sad, right? We will come back to that. The next question, can we support one another to achieve our goals and honour our values? Larry may feel that he is where he wants to be. He is happy, he is content, he is okay with spending the rest of his life this way, but you want to grow and of course you would like to grow together. But can he support you and honour your desire for spiritual growth? He doesn't disparage it or shame you does he?
No. I don't think he shames me. I think he is a bit condescending at times about it, I mean I don't talk about it to be honest with you. I don't really talk about it with him because if I do, [that goes] down like a lead balloon. He is not disparaging but he is condescending at times or can be jokey with something that is important to me, so I let it go.
I wonder if his jokiness is a defence against some of those more delicate, more moving emotions that create a sense of vulnerability?
Absolutely, absolutely. It's a defence mechanism. but there are so many defence mechanisms that I am just tired. And I feel a bit like, what's the point?
You don't feel secure it seems in his support?
(sighs) That is a really hard question to answer because Larry would encourage me, support me to do anything. [She gives a series of examples about how he would support her in practical ways, then moves to emotional support. She describes a glowing review and endorsement.] I said to Larry, 'Oh, do you want to read this, what someone has written?' and he was like, 'No, not really.' I said, 'It's only about 200 words. It will take you about five minutes to read.' and he was like, 'Oh, just tell me the gist of it.' and then his reaction to that will be something like, 'Oh another story about you being amazing.'
Oh really?
Yeah
Okay that's a -
'I'm only joking, I'm only joking. Oh that's really nice, that is really nice.' He likes it like, [tells of other endorsements from clients] so I told Larry that, and he loves that kind of stuff, cause it almost feels that it gives him some kudos, you know? He likes it that his wife is successful and doing well. He likes those stories on one level, but also can't really cope with them in terms of me being amazing. He likes it in the context of our relationship, but feels very threatened by it. Like, 'No-one ever tells me I am amazing.'
Well, do you think he is amazing?

I think there are a lot of elements of Larry that I absolutely do think are amazing, absolutely do, you know? Many things I think he is amazing in and there are other areas of Larry that I think he is an absolute twat.

Ahh, bless your heart.

Really bad, isn't it? And I do, I get the absolute ick from certain things he does. I'm like. 'Aah, like this is so.'

Well, it might be worth talking about what those things are, because, in terms of you being able to get out of the relationship what you want, I have some suggestions. But let's keep going, before I start trying to jump in and fix it, and find out what's going on there. So, he is supportive but with, with a little bit of resentment thrown in?

Yeah, I would say so.

Or jealousy perhaps?

Jealousy.

Yeah. Feeling worth-less-than you are.

Definitely.

And of course, the direction I am going to go is supporting him, letting him know that you appreciate him, and appreciate his support. But let's get onto the next: Are we able to continue to evolve and mature over time together? And that sounds crucial.

See that's where I am, that's where I am stuck, because I don't know the answer to that question and my gut instinct is 'no.'

Well …

But, having said, 'No,' I do think that he has a massive potential for that to be a 'yes,' but he is stuck. He is so stuck Charley. He is so stuck and his sense of reflection and openness is shutting down. I can feel that's what has happened in the last twelve months. He is less reflective about what happens. He will not talk about stuff in the same way that we used to talk about things. It's like his ego has got weaker over time. There have been a couple of instances over the last couple of weeks that have massively upset him. He hasn't realised that they have massively upset other people too

Really?

Or maybe he has but he doesn't know how to repair it. [She tells about an incident between Larry and their children that escalated with hurt feelings all around.] But I, the person I am worrying most about in this situation is him, cause I know what is going on for him is huge. He has gone upstairs feeling really shit about himself and his ego is so, it feels like it's quite fragile. Our daughter is nineteen. She has got issues like any kid has but within an hour she is alright and she has calmed down. But with him, he will internalise all of that. The next morning he didn't stay a word so I knew that he was still really upset. [Later] I sent him a message saying, 'Are you okay? I am really worried about you.'

mm

now I am worried about him because he is not talking about it, he is not talking to me about what happened whereas normally he would, and I said, so he said erm, err, he said 'I'm just in a funk I can't seem to shift it, but I will be okay I always am, I certainly don't want to talk about it.' And then I said 'just remember, just remember that erm, err just remember that it's only because everyone loves you so much that they get upset,' and he said, 'it doesn't feel like it sometimes I feel obsolete and not very important, my opinion is never needed or wanted,' and then he talks about [another event with another of their children and their girlfriend resulting in hurt feelings all around.]

Mm, dear, well ...

The issue was that Larry couldn't talk to me about it. And this is new. This has only happened in the last twelve months that he just can't talk or reflect on stuff. This is my biggest problem. It's not the incidents that happen. There have always been instances like this but he has always been able to reflect and think and learn and now it just feels like he's gone 'I have done enough now. You don't fucking love me for who I am' like his big statement is, 'that's who I am' kind of 'leave me alone' kind of thing why do I have to change all the time?

Well err, yeah and, and I, and I think that is the crux of the problem: 'you don't love me for who I am,' his perception of that. Whoa! Right, I'm going to bookmark this for right now and come back to it. 'Are we able to give ourselves shared meaning in life?'

Yes probably

Okay okay. Is that enough on that you feel confident in that?

Yeah in bigger picture stuff yes.

Okay, and the next question is, can we take satisfaction from our partner's achievements?

Yes.

Okay and does Larry take satisfaction in your achievements?

I think so.

That's good. now we come down to the next level, esteem: how we feel about self and others? How do you feel about Larry when you are with him? When you are interacting with him?

How do I feel about him?

Yeah.

Can I feel all sorts of things?

Okay, want to name a few?

I feel anxious.

Okay.

I feel disappointed

Oh dear. Okay

I feel love, huge amounts of love.

Okay, okay.

yeah.

And err how do you feel about yourself? When you are with Larry?

Erm? How do I feel about myself?

Yes.

(sighs) Invisible. No, that's a bit harsh. I am not invisible err, how do I feel when I am with Larry? Err? Bored.

Bored? Wow okay.

Or how do I feel about me? Was that the question, how do I feel about me?

Yeah, yourself?

What do I feel about me?

Yeah so when you are bored, how do you feel about yourself?

Erm? I don't know, I don't know what the feeling is, the thought is that I have kind of let myself down in, I am letting myself down

Okay.

But I don't know what the feeling is then. Like a bit, kind of embarrassed maybe. I don't know? Err?

Okay, this is huge now. Embarrassed, so letting yourself down by being with Larry?

Yeah.

Okay wow, okay okay okay.

Like I am betraying myself.

Yeah. I get it. Erm? Well, I don't want to overplay that but we may have just hit the you know the key here.

Nail on the head.

Yeah yeah and err digging a little deeper when you, when you perceive yourself as betraying yourself then how do you feel about yourself?

(sighs) just like I am letting myself down really like it could be better than this.

okay okay. Erm, yeah okay. Um, again if we take those as messages you are giving yourself what's the feeling that goes with it? I could do better, I'm …

I am thinking sadness, I think that is where the sadness is.

Okay err alright, so we'll stick with sadness there. How does Larry feel about you when he is with you? You know what is your impression of that?

See I think he feels inferior when he is with me.

mm, mm

I think he feels not good enough, that's how he feels.

Yeah exactly err, and

That's the, it's such an issue here because this is all attachment, I think this is all attachment stuff.

You do?

It's not about me, and so because I have got that kind of insight, I get what's going on for him but he doesn't, and so what do you do with that? Because like I don't think for him it would be any different no matter who he was with he would feel something—unless, maybe unless he was with someone who he saw not as bright as him or you know something like that, but then I don't think he would be content with somebody who wasn't very bright or politically aware you know, that would be a massive issue for him. I think if he was asked, 'how do you feel when you are with Sue?' he would say, 'Well sometimes I don't feel good enough.' He has said to me, 'I feel disappointed in the relationship,' and I think he would be able to articulate that to you. He would be able to say, 'I don't feel good enough for Sue and I feel that she is disappointed me in all the time.'

mm okay

But that's horrible that he feels like that and I think that's why I think 'oh you know what maybe I am not the right person for him,' you know? [She describes some very bad events from his childhood that she believes contribute to his shame.] This man carries huge amounts of shame. When you hear those kind of stories you think, 'Well, do you know what, this is the part of Larry that I think is amazing.' you know I think he is an amazing person given his start in life.

mm mm

You know, this man who started being treated absolutely appallingly, being absolutely terrified that his dad was going to kill his mum on a daily basis and going to kill him and being shamed for something that clearly was to do with terror, you know? And then you get this man who is reflective and thoughtful and open, and cares about oppression, cares about the world politically, is able to maintain relationships, is able to really invest in his relationship with his kids. He is an amazing person and that's what makes this so hard.

Well, so

But it's not like he is my project, do you know? He can't be my project.

Well, I am going to suggest that I am not sure you have a lot of choice if you want it to be different. I may not understand what you mean by your 'project.'

It's not my job to rescue him it's not my job to fix him.

No it's not but it's [your choice, I opine. Then we go on to the questions about commitment at the love and belonging level]: Are you will-

ing to make a commitment? You have already done that. What risk am I willing to take? I suppose that actually is a good question: What risk are you willing to take now with and for Larry? I think the big challenge is being honest about where you are. There was a point where you were saying how you felt, 'Oh, I think I could do better. I'm embarrassed.' I think that's probably coming through to him, and it seems to me the two of you are in a negative feedback spiral, yeah?
Yeah.
And the obvious way to reverse that is, do the opposite.
I guess that's what I was trying to do, by saying to him, 'I am worried about you,' and saying to him, 'We all really love you,' when actually what I wanted to say is, 'You behaved like a twat and you know you need to apologise to our daughter.'
[A discussion of ways to handle communicating her dissatisfaction]
We have hit on the key now: shame. When you see things through that shame filter you are being defensive. The triple F [freeze, fight, flight] is operating and all you can see is the threat.
Yeah.
[More discussion about Larry and whether he will accept help.]
I am going to challenge you, cause you are doing the typical C thing, I think, of stating what you want in the form of a complaint about not getting it. If you can do the translator I recommend to avoidant men who are in relationship with women using a C strategy: learn to translate this complaint into a request for something positive. So, because I am not working with Larry, I am working with you, the challenge is with you. [Discussing how to make a criticism into a complaint, and a complaint into a request.]
Everything is a criticism. If you have a different opinion than him, he hears it as a criticism.
Mm okay so that's his filter and I think all you can do with that is point that out to him, you know? That is why the second part of the 'I feel ... when ... because ....' model is *essential*. If you don't use that, 'what I heard you say ...' you can't know what he is hearing and how it is different from what you are saying.
Yeah.
It's easy to ask, 'Hey, hang on. What did you hear me say?' And he might come out with something like, 'Well, you think I am a real piece of shit and you are sorry you married me.' Well, no, that's not it and ... You just have to confront that. Has this helped?
Yeah, it's helped to unpick it. But with these conversations I always come back to the same point: that it's me that has to do something different and I am just a bit tired of that. I am a bit tired of not being with a grown up.

Yeah, I get what you are saying, I understand.
Anyway, the biggest thing for me, for next time, I just feel like I am not brave enough to leave him.
That was the next thing: the vulnerability and acceptance level. There are more questions here that we need to ask. And the other unsaid question is, which way are you going to go with it?

I thought as we were going through this that Sue would take this new ordering of information and use it to good effect. She did. She and Larry had an open and honest discussion about how they were feeling, their needs, and how to go about getting them met. The relationships have been repaired with the children as well. Fingers crossed, they will keep going in this new direction.

TECHNIQUES FOR WORKING WITH FAMILIES

Crittenden and Dallos have written concerning the integration of family dynamics in working with attachment.[6] Crittenden and Landini have written of the 'functional family formulation,' and they and their colleagues have been developing this model for some years. The most exciting development that I have found recently is a new approach to working with families that is being pioneered by Dr. Rudi Dallos and Dr. Ben Grey. Rudi and Arlene Vetere's ANT was introduced in Chap. 2 and has accompanied us throughout our journey. Dr. Grey and Dr. Steve Farnfield have created the Meaning of the Child (MotC[7]) interview. This is an interview of the parent regarding their relationship with their child. It is similar to the AAI, and overlaps somewhat so that if the parent's AAI has not been done, it gives the MotC coder some understanding of the parent's attachment strategy. Drs Dallos and Grey have taken this a step further. They are developing the Systemic MotC, which is taking the concept of Systemic Family Therapy as adapted in ANT and combining it with the MotC. The purpose is to move beyond the dyadic study of attachment, as reflected in the AAI, and develop a systemic study of attachment. I commend their efforts and am pleased to be able to explore this with them. All these are based wholly or partly on Dr. Crittenden's Dynamic Maturational Model of attachment.

Adlerian Family Therapy

Adler's approach to family therapy was rather elaborate, using multifamily groups with both an outer and an inner circle, with more experienced families serving as guides for the newcomers. Adler also introduced the concept of the birth order factor, which is another feature that we have not yet factored in and the effect of siblings in the family dynamic. I am aware that children in families often follow the pattern of hero, scapegoat, lost child, and mascot, respectively. There have been various explanations for why that particular order, and they don't always occur in that order. As that has been written about extensively elsewhere[8] I will not go into it here. There have been various approaches to this.[9] Limitations of time and space do not allow us to explore these further in this book.

Addiction and Families

In the addiction treatment field, we have been addressing these issues for decades. The primary factor in whether or not someone overcomes addictive disorders is how good is their support network, and the primary factor in a support network is family support. Conversely, if someone has a subversive family system, they may need to get away from them in order to have a healthy recovery. The family system is very likely implicated in the origins of the addictive disorder, and so whether they will be a help or a hindrance in recovery is an important consideration.

As a human being who has gone through much of what is described in this book, I have experienced the intersectionality of abuse and dysfunctional family relationships. The Adult Children of Alcoholics (ACOA) movement and the Al-Anon (co-dependents of alcoholics) and Alateen (children of alcoholics) movements and the various 12-step spin-off groups have recognized the impact of abuse and neglect on families. We have long been aware of the impact of family dynamics on the individuals and the impact of individual dysfunction on the family. These 12-step approaches are valuable, even lifesaving, for many. Yet they are also very hit or miss, depending on how well each individual can fit into the model.

I have also observed that even when the 12-step model is successful at suppressing a particular additive disorder, the underlying need remains unmet and so the disorder migrates to another realm: the alcoholic who succeeds in getting sober from alcohol, but who becomes a '13th-stepper,' the term denoting someone who hits on newcomers into the programme; or who suicides after decades of 'recovery.'

In working with families, I would ideally like to have AAIs from the parents, other assessments such as the School Age Assessment,[10] the Transition to Adulthood Attachment Interview (the AAI adapted for late teens and early adulthood), the MotC, and of course any other instrument that is useful. As one may imagine, this could quickly escalate into unmanageability because we are having to juggle the application of resources and possibilities in the best possible manner. It is a challenge.

It was Adler who identified that the worst parenting situation for the child is to have one parent who is indulgent and another who is authoritarian. We can compare this to the child who has parents using two different attachment strategies, an A and a C. This means that with one parent, say for example, a depressed A+ mother, the child needs to adopt a C strategy for their optimal outcome. It takes escalation and persistence for the child to get mom's attention and have some hope of getting their needs met. If dad is C+, using guilt to 'seduce' (not in a sexual sense but in getting compliance) or anger to intimidate, then to escalate risks blurring of boundaries and conflict. The child then finds an A strategy of compulsive compliance to be adaptive. Great, we might think, the child has both strategies available: the best of both worlds. It is more likely to be the worst of both worlds, because the information processing is distorted in different ways. While the combination of strategies can useful when blended into a B type response, this is not what insecure attachment creates. It is, however, a possibility that we can use to enable clients to reorganize by consciously choosing which elements of the strategy to emphasize and which to correct.

The books that I rely on are those in the Adlerian tradition: *Children: the Challenge*[11] and *Raising a Responsible Child*,[12] Gottman's book, *Raising an Emotionally Intelligent Child*,[13] and two books about indigenous parenting: *Hunt, Gather, Parent*[14] and *The Continuum Concept*.[15] These books all rely on the same proposition that children need to develop in their own way; that raising a child is virtually impossible to do successfully alone—it really does take a village, metaphorically speaking of course; and that our job is to keep them safe and provide the 'scaffolding' to help them build themselves.

Notes

1. Gottman, J. (2018). *The seven principles for making marriage work.* Hachette UK.
2. Gottman, J. M. (1976). A couple's guide to communication. *(No Title).*
3. Notarius, C., & Markman, H. (1993). *We can work it out: Making sense of marital conflict.* Putnam Adult.
4. Watzlawick, P., & Jackson, D. D. (2010). On human communication (1964). *Journal of Systemic Therapies, 29*(2), 53–68.
5. Notarius, C., & Markman, H. (1993). *We can work it out: Making sense of marital conflict.* Putnam Adult.
6. Crittenden, P. M., & Dallos, R. (2009). All in the family: Integrating attachment and family systems theories. *Clinical Child Psychology and Psychiatry, 14*(3), 389–409.
7. Grey, B., & Farnfield, S. (2017). The Meaning of the Child Interview: A new procedure for assessing and understanding parent–child relationships of 'at-risk' families. *Clinical child psychology and psychiatry, 22*(2), 204–218.
8. Woititz, J. G. (1990). *Adult children of alcoholics: Expanded edition.* Health Communications, Inc.; Black, C. (2020). *It will never happen to me: Growing up with addiction as youngsters, adolescents, and adults.* Central Recovery Press.
9. Maabreh, S. M., Faiez, F., Al-Kousheh, M., & Maabarha, S. (2020). The effectiveness of a counseling program based on the model of Virginia Satir in improving quality of life and reducing negative communication patterns among a sample of wives in Irbid governorate. *Res. Humanit. Soc. Sci, 10*, 84–96.; Olson, D. H. (2000). Circumplex model of marital and family systems. *Journal of family therapy, 22*(2), 144–167.
10. Crittenden, P., Robson, K., & Tooby, A. (2015). Validation of the School-age Assessment of Attachment in a short-term longitudinal study. *Clinical Child Psychology and Psychiatry, 20*(3), 348–365.
11. Dreikurs, R., & Stolz, V. (1991). *Children: the Challenge: The Classic Work on Improving Parent-Child Relations—Intelligent, Humane, and Eminently Practical.* Penguin.
12. Dinkmeyer, D. C., McKay, G. D., & Dinkmeyer, D. (1996). *Raising a responsible child: How to prepare your child for today's complex world.* Simon and Schuster.
13. Gottman, J. (2011). *Raising an emotionally intelligent child.* Simon and Schuster.
14. Doucleff, M. (2021). *Hunt, gather, parent: What ancient cultures can teach us about the lost art of raising happy, helpful little humans.* Simon and Schuster.
15. Liedloff, J. (2004). *The continuum concept.* Penguin UK.

CHAPTER 9

Creating New Narratives

One of the first things that I noticed when working through AAI transcripts with clients was their adherence to a narrative. Often when I read the first part of the clients' answer to a question, if I paused, they would pick up the narrative from the point where I had stopped and carry on with the narrative, as if reading from a script. In some cases it would be virtually word for word. In all cases it would be a very similar narrative. I was surprised by this. Not so much that it occurred, but the power of it. Once started, it was as if they were compelled by some force to finish the narrative. This usually occurred in the earlier parts of the interview.

I was equally surprised in the opposite direction. With some clients, when we got to the last third of the interview where the reflective, integrative questions are located, clients would make comments such as 'Oh, I would never answer that question that way now.' They had reorganized and had created a new narrative. Typically, I would ask them how they would answer it today. They would then give me a balanced, coherent narrative explaining how they saw their parents, their motivations, and what they had learned from the experience that would be useful going forward. In short, they had created a new narrative that was more coherent and more useful. I have not chosen those to use here. Rather, I have chosen clients, all of whom you have met before, who have struggled to break out of the old narrative and who have persisted, practised, and are achieving

© The Author(s), under exclusive license to Springer Nature Switzerland AG 2024
C. Shults, *Attachment Centred Therapy*, Palgrave Texts in Counselling and Psychotherapy,
https://doi.org/10.1007/978-3-031-60851-3_9

new narratives for themselves. They had the courage to face their fears and go through the process of change, where old ways are challenged before new ways have developed sufficiently to replace them. You have to quit going down the old pathway in order to create a new one.

In relating these stories, I have included some excerpts from transcripts of sessions. As usual, I have edited these quite heavily due to the limitations of space and to hold your interest. The emphasis is on the point that I wish to make. It is not done to deceive you or to make me look better (although, regrettably, it often does). Feel free to imagine all sorts of 'ums,' 'uhs,' and other dysfluency as needed.

GREGORY'S WALKING HOLIDAY

Gregory, whom we met in the dream section, and Patty, his partner, were going on a walking holiday. Because his fitness level was better than Patty's, Gregory had put some effort into planning walks they could both do and enjoy. Gregory likes to plan things carefully and gets very upset when things don't go the way he has planned them. Patty is flexible about planning, to the point of regularly being late and disorganized. If one believes in a higher power, one might surmise that they have been put together intentionally to get them both to moderate their extreme positions in this regard!

Gregory starts the session describing the difficulty:

> I've got quite a bit to relate, really, about the weekend that we went on. It was a bit of a mixed weekend. Erm, some difficulties with Patty and mainly sort of, self-inflicted erm difficulties. Quite alarming, really, how I continue to get [upset] over experiences with Patty, and I feel bad about it. In fact, it got to a state on Saturday night, when I was thinking to myself, in all conscience, I should say to Patty, 'Look, I'm sorry, but you know I, I can't erm, offer you that, err love and support that erm you are entitled to.' Looking back, these were no big deal on Patty's part. So Patty said one or two things on one or two occasions which seriously affected me but when I play them back to myself, or you, we will find that in fact that there is really no big deal, you know? What's all the fuss about?

This is excellent self-reflection on Gregory's part. He had planned walks that would not be too taxing for Patty. He was then quite upset when Patty suggested that they go on an easy walk that a stranger had told them about. Here is his version of events:

Anyway, on Saturday morning I said to Patty, 'It would be nice to go to these places that I'd mentioned,' and Patty said to me, 'I thought we could go to this viaduct that this fella was talking about last night,' and I was sort of—just, 'That's it' … I was massively taken aback, by her—bit more than idea—this sort of erm, this plan to go to this place that this fella had mentioned where it hadn't previously been discussed as a possibility.

He then relates how he had 'mentioned' this to Patty several times. The mildness which he relates in mentioning this walks is in sharp contrast to his comment:

I was furious with her about this. Erm, quite why I had such an extreme reaction I don't know. If that had been delivered with a little less colour than it was on my part then that would have been a perfectly satisfactory response and end of story,

He then relates how they compromised and went on the walk he had planned that day and the impromptu walk on the following day. Next, they were going to visit a village, and it involved Gregory driving and Patty map-reading, typically a time for conflict between them, disagreement about where to sit for a picnic, and so on. As previously, Gregory is focused, not on his annoyance with Patty so much as his annoyance with himself:

The affect was amplified. I was very irritated with her when she was map reading and whether we went the wrong way, just getting more annoyed than was appropriate. And, yeah, so it, it, was erm, very disappointing and you know I was thinking, 'Well, of course one should be able to … say to Patty, you know, 'I am feeling blah blah because of, you know when you said, I felt when you said blah blah,' but unfortunately … *[Here Gregory is referring to the 'I feel … when … because …' model for expressing feelings, which he knows, but was unable to do at the time. Conscious Incompetence]* And you know it took me a day or two to compute really what was going on, why I felt as strongly as I did.

Gregory is frustrated that he cannot understand why he over-reacts.

I said, 'I am just going for a walk up the hills now.' And the best part of the day was me pacing on my own up a hill near the house and it was in fact fabulous. It was a beautiful evening. Saw the sun go down over the Lakeland tops, it was just beautiful.

Notice the missing 'I' and the description of enjoying the walk all by himself, both indicative of the A6 Compulsive Self-reliance strategy. He then reflects:

> I feel bad, sort of, recounting these things to be honest, erm, but it, you know and I—I should of course be able at some stage to be able to talk to Patty about some of these things—to apologise really erm, one more unfortunate incident erm so again on the Sunday you know—gosh I don't know it's—I do feel as I say I do feel bad recounting these things.

There follows a discussion of their drive back and some of Patty's background, triggered by a particular village, that Gregory was very sympathetic in relating. Gregory also shares his discomfort about some of Patty's personal idiosyncrasies that may be partly cultural. He then plans how he can speak to Patty about his over-reaction:

> Okay, how do I talk about what went on? ... I just have to say something like, 'Patty, I am sorry about how I overreacted to you on a couple of occasions in Yorkshire,' and not, again not justify it in any way but just to, to—perhaps explain what was going on in my head and just reassure her that, you know, I didn't hold her responsible for what she had said and that my reaction was, you know wholly inappropriate, and erm, erm. I don't—yeah so full stop really erm, yeah so anyway over to you I think Charley.
> **Well Gregory I mean that's err quite a lot. Let me share with you first what I was thinking. Err I don't know, maybe last night maybe this morning, was of, of reassuring you. I don't know that you need my reassurance, but I just wanted to comment that I think you and Patty are going to make it. I mean fingers crossed. I see you lift your eyebrows at that comment. (chuckles) Are you surprised?**
> Well, erm, erm um, I am not sure really Charley I don't know. I know what I feel.
> **Maybe. Not sure that's a good thing or a bad thing huh? (laughing)**
> Yeah.
> **Yeah. I was just thinking, because you're engaged in a process and you are making progress, it's as simple as that. You have gotten through the worst part. It's just going to start getting better now. And of course, when I have thoughts like that sometimes I always question myself, 'Oh, am I getting that right,' you know? What you are sharing this morning is really great. It's full of promise and also actuation. Because the questions you are asking yourself, the comments, the whole way**

you are framing it, is your quest to be able to understand and deal better with Patty, and also recognising that your reactions are a bit over the top. Sometimes *way* over the top! And you feel badly about it so you are motivated to change it. I think it's important that at the same time you are feeling badly about the behaviour that you are not feeling badly about yourself, because you have been dedicated to changing things and you have worked steadily toward it. So I think that you are in a position to do some really good work with Patty, working on the relationship, relating and that's what we will do right now.

We then proceed to process what had happened, how he might have handled it differently, and preparing to do so using, first, the REBT method to check out that his beliefs are rational and to change them if not. Then we go on to using the 'I feel … when … because …' model to express those feelings. Then we look at the effect that some have written about popularly[1] and some humorously,[2] and some more scientifically[3]:

> I sometimes say to myself, 'Patty is from another planet.' I think to myself, 'Patty lives a parallel life to me and.'
> **And that is exactly right. It's not literally correct, a different planet, but it is a whole different territory and err if you can, can you remember that? Can you accept that and love her anyway?**
> Yes err of course, of course I could. I would accept that I'm unduly erm, don't know what the word is, but sort of matter of fact and rationalist and yeah and—and I can see Patty sees things differently yeah.
> **Yeah. I imagine, I am trying to imagine myself in your situation. I imagine it would have hurt your feelings.**
> Hurt my feelings? Erm, like, very disappointed that she doesn't want to do what I had planned to do.

I then go on to further empathize with his feelings. Notice how, in the previous dialogue, he doesn't endorse hurt feelings but switches it to a more cognitive 'disappointed.' All his planning was worth less than the suggestion from a stranger in a pub. This worth-less-ness triggered Gregory's shame. I referred to a session some time ago when we went through his AAI a second time and counted 29 instances of shame. Gregory doesn't immediately agree with the shame suggestion.

> **And that's why you get so annoyed. That's why it comes out with this vehement quality. Does that make sense?**

It does make sense, and it's quite affecting to me, the thought of what that might have been ... and erm, yeah, surprised in a way that I wasn't able to, erm, feel that. You know, to experience that sense of shame that you—or sense of worth less ness that erm, you are describing, but yeah.
I think that when you experience these intrusions of negative affect, the defensive position is so strong that you get that immediate reaction—kaboom! And it's already occupied your mind, and because of the way you function it stayed with you for days.
I can't know that what you are suggesting is a real prompt for my reaction. I suspect, I suspect it is, and I suspect erm, my sort of erm, almost, almost shock at your suggestion, and the—emotional impact it's having is, you know would suggest it's pretty close to the mark yeah. *[This is the 'shock of recognition.']*

We reached the limit of Gregory's ZPD in this session! He is not going to try to communicate with Patty what he has mentally rehearsed in this session. Still, he has accomplished a lot: (1) he focuses on himself, not Patty, as the source of the problem; (2) he recognizes that he had an opportunity to use a new behaviour and share his feelings and reasoning with Patty; (3) he then practises doing so; (4) he accepts my suggestion that it is shame that is causing him to react the way he does; (5) he experiences the shock of recognition; (6) he describes strong affective arousal as a result; (7) he rehearses actually sharing with Patty his thoughts and feelings, even though he decides he is not yet ready to do that.

We did not directly address, though it is apparent in this session, that Gregory is preoccupied with getting things right and performing a task. That gets in the way of him enjoying relationships for their own sake.

Gregory had another dream recently. He referred to it as a 'dream image,' but upon examination, it seems to be more than that. This dream involved his mother, who, as best I recall, had not previously made an appearance in Gregory's dreams. I thought that was significant in itself, since the main blockage of Gregory's memories seems to concern his mother. In this dream, he was cleaning a vessel made of glass. It was cylindrical, with straight sides (he first described it as 'a little bowl'). It was dirty inside. He thought that he had cleaned 'a ring on the inside of this bowl.' 'I said to my mother, "I've cleaned this a bit", and looked at it and she said, "Well, no, you haven't."' He looked and it was still 'murky and grubby.' He didn't recall any particular feelings. 'My mother wasn't aggressive or scornful. I was feeling more puzzled than put down or angry or anything.'

My interpretation of this dream is that it is consistent with the artist and the accountant dream. The vessel that he was cleaning is consistent with his inner self, his soul, or his spirit. This is a theme that recurs with many clients, of a feeling of emptiness inside. The 'hole in the soul.' In recovery work, that emptiness is filled by becoming who you really are. As e.e. cummings put it:

> It takes courage to grow up
> and become
> who you really are.

I imagined that Gregory's mother had appeared to let him know that it was okay to have a hard look at their relationship, hence the glass container that he was trying to clean. But he still has more work to do because his efforts to clean 'a ring on the inside' were insufficient according to his mother, and he had to agree when he looked again. However, he has made progress. This dream represents the progress, with the image of his mother encouraging him. This gives Gregory permission and encouragement to clear away more of the 'murky grubbiness' that prevents his seeing clearly what is inside the vessel. This is the same information that is missing in the artist and accountant dream.

In addition, Gregory is now considering taking the plunge, sort of, by wading in a little deeper by buying Patty a ring for Christmas. An expensive ring, one that she will pick out with him, but without declaring that it is an engagement ring. Not yet, anyway.

ANDREA AND THE MEN IN HER LIFE

With Andrea, the client with whom I opened this book, her AAI had revealed a family history of trauma, her own attachment trauma, struggle to survive, emotionally, of sexual abuse, spiritual abuse, and emotional abuse. At this point in therapy, we had worked through a lot together.

I had a pretty good idea of what Andrea's childhood had been like. Her mother had been stressed to the max, struggling to make ends meet on their hardscrabble farm. Andrea was the third child of four, with a brother ten years older and sister eight years older, and a sister two years younger. We knew from history related by her older sister that mother had little time for Andrea. She usually communicated with her through Andrea's older siblings. Andrea's memory of her childhood was vague.

The parts she did remember weren't pleasant. Sharing a bedroom with her taciturn and bitter grandmother, sometimes with mom. Sitting on her father's knee when she was four years old, before he left to go to another country to work to make money to support the family, where he stayed through most of her childhood, only occasionally visiting for seasonal holidays. She told a story of her sister, left to watch Andrea by mother, who, wanting to go outside to play, turned the bassinet upside down with Andrea restrained underneath. Her sister had told her that one.

Mother was distant and depressed. She worked daily on their farm outside the village and lived in fear of not having enough to eat. She had survived World War II, though she had been raped in the process. Grandmother had survived World War I.

She recounted six events of childhood sexual abuse by relatives, friends of the family, and strangers. None of them were penetrative. All were intrusive. She told of them casually, without emotion, as if each had been an ordinary experience. At the same time that the men of her village were approaching her sexually, she was being conditioned negatively towards sex by her family. This was reinforced by the Catholic Church which dominated the village. The women of the village gossiped and shamed girls and women who were 'loose' sexually. The church was condemning and shaming about any sexuality outside of marriage. Her brother, ten years older, repeatedly reminded her, at their mother's urging, that any woman who enjoyed sex was certain to become a prostitute, the most shameful thing imaginable.

Against this background, Andrea was left to learn about sex and relationships with men on her own. It did not go well.

It began with a married man. She was actually living in the home of the family for the summer to help the mother take care of their children. The father came on to her repeatedly. He would come into her bedroom in the evenings. She experienced his attention with a mix of emotions: flattered, that he should find her interesting; fear, of sexual involvement because she knew it was 'wrong' by the standards of her family and her strongly Catholic community; confusion, because this man was a fine, upstanding member of the church and the community, and they were in his home, in her bedroom; more fear because of the possibility of them being discovered by the man's wife; excitement, because he was attractive and his attention to her caused her to feel special and important; shame, because of what her brother had told her about sexual excitement and pleasure leading to prostitution; last of all, she felt powerful, because she realized that she could use sex to gain power with men.

Next, she had a liaison with an unmarried man who was about ten years older. She would meet him in the village, then they would drive to a remote location in the mountains to make out. Soon she left the village to attend college, and she used sex as a way to have relationships. She went through a series of relationships that started, lasted a year or two, and then ended. But Andrea always made sure she had another relationship to go to before she left the one that she was in. She carried on this way through graduate school and then post-graduate professional training and into her profession. Then, when she was in her late 30s, she became pregnant. She decided that if she ever wanted to have a child, the time was now. She married the man who had gotten her pregnant and moved to his country of origin.

Andrea was referred to me by another therapist. Her presenting issue was her relationship with her husband, with whom she had one child, a daughter. Both she and her husband were successful professionals who worked together, but her husband had all the financial control. She described their sex life as if she was his real live sex doll. She had learned that it was easier to just say yes and let him use her for sex even though she never enjoyed it. Andrea's memory of her early childhood was sparse. This suggested to me a possible switch of attachment strategies for her later years. I assessed her attachment strategy as being A5–6.

As for her relationship with me and a degree of dependence, I did not discourage this. I surmised that Andrea was relating to me as a transitional attachment figure. This allowed me to play that role in terms of her treatment. She trusted me and took what I had to say to heart. The danger was that she would move deeper into her A+ strategy into A7–8: Delusional Idealization and Externally Assembled Self. I was aware of this possibility and used it to continue to encourage her to move towards the B3 strategy and to trust her feelings more. As she became more affectively expressive, she moves *towards* the C side of the model. This was the basis of the A7–8. The emotion of trust and excitement about the new learnings she was getting were what propelled her in the C direction, but this was only a *direction* of movement. At the same time, as her distortions of information, affective and cognitive, were eliminated, this moved her higher up the model, *towards* B3.

In our first meetings, at her request we sat at a table in the foyer of my home/office. She was quite rigid, sitting bolt upright, always well-dressed, and took copious notes.

Her relationship with her husband continued to deteriorate as we worked together. I recommended reading *We Can Work It Out*[4] and *The Seven Principles for Making Marriage Work*.[5] Despite Andrea being a dedicated student, these books did not help her to save her marriage. To the contrary, they highlighted what was wrong with it. Her husband never came to a therapy session, so I never met him.

Having reluctantly entered into marriage, motivated by her pregnancy, Andrea now reluctantly considered dissolving her marriage. This was complicated by their daughter having an eating disorder. At Andrea's request, I met with the daughter, Racine, on a few occasions. They also attended a specialist eating disorder outpatient treatment programme. Fortunately, Racine responded well to the treatment programme and went from being seriously malnourished to being a normal weight. However, as is often the case with addictive disorders, even though the identified behaviour is extinguished by a treatment programme or some other intervention, the same dynamic emerges in a different, sometimes more destructive, way. For Racine, this became sex and drugs.

As they went through the family meeting component of Racine's treatment, Andrea was able to see her husband's attitude in stark relief. She realized that he considered it an inconvenience to have to attend the meetings. He regarded the problem as having nothing to do with him. Never mind that his criticism and control towards Racine were a significant feature in the aetiology of her illness: commenting on her weight (too much), how much food she was eating (too much), and her academic performance (not enough) all contributed to Racine's perception that she was not good enough (shame) and her preoccupation with food restriction and weight loss to have some control and to please her father.

Andrea was also determined to do 'the right thing,' consistent with her A4 strategy. The higher strategies, such as A6, generally include the lesser strategies. She had to spend a considerable amount of time and emotional effort in order to make ending the marriage 'the right thing to do,' contrary to the teachings of the Catholic Church. Eventually she got up the courage to do so. Racine was pleased.

After a period of readjustment, to include sorting out their enmeshed financial arrangements, Andrea and I discussed her relationship status, and she decided to try dating again. She turned to the internet as a way to meet potential partners.

Depending on your experiences with internet dating, you might be thinking, 'Oh dear!' You would be quite right to do so. Andrea was naïve and trusting. She was a good student and she learned quickly, relatively speaking. Learning takes longer as we get older. It's not that we can't grasp the ideas as we get older, it's that the behavioural and emotional changes that the new ideas call for take far longer to become encoded in our neurology as the default pathway: the new 'pathway through the forest.'[6]

I was surprised when she told me of some of her exploits which I understood as sexual promiscuity. This is not so surprising when we remember that the A5 strategy of Compulsive Promiscuity is located next to the A6 strategy of Compulsive Self-reliance. It also, on reflection, was consistent with what she had told me of her earlier experiences with men, and how she had learned that she could use sex with men to get the comfort, companionship, and approval that she craved.

People using an A strategy discount or 'avoid' their own negative emotions. They tend to attribute any deficiencies to themselves. They also tend to suppress information that creates negative feelings. Thus, they can be gullible. The following story is an example of what I mean. They act out of shame, the sense of unworthiness, and so they believe that they have to 'do something' to 'earn' the love and approval of others.

In order to recover, we have to challenge those erroneous beliefs. During this process, Andrea sent me the following email:

> Dear Charley
> I have reflected about our last session. I have become aware that, despite my wish *not* to repeat with Helios what I have done with Edward and other men, I have fallen in the same trap: giving sex to receive affection. It did not work and I found myself lonely and sad for having lied to him.
>
> As a start, I would like to tell the truth and write Helios a letter. With your agreement I would like you to look at it and make it understandable. I have in mind when you helped me with the most recent letter to Edward about the money he owes me. It was *so* clear that he gave me the money back. I call it the language that men understand. I feel I speak the language that women but not men understand. I am trying to learn the "male" language. Not sure I can succeed.

Sadly, I have no hopes that Helios or whoever can understand my reasons, and I feel ashamed the only language that I know to keep a man close to me is sex. Can you teach me other languages? Tell me why I have learned it? What I dislike most is that I try to give men orgasms so that I can be left in peace. I have this thought that a man can emotionally and physically hurt if he has not received his sexual dose.

Sex is my enemy. Still, I use it, and well, apparently. But it is not genuine which makes me feel guilty for doing something against my principles.

You are right, I have the Catholic idea of wanting to be immaculate and conceive without sex, which is not natural, you tell me. But I find it very difficult to accept that mother nature has made us to have sex to guarantee reproduction and survival.

I feel shame and inferior that I can't say 'no' but have no idea when to say yes.

Looking at the future, I have considered going ahead in my life without sex, enjoy Racine, and wait for grandchildren to come and so on, as you said today. It would be the immaculate route.

At the same time I like the closeness, warmth and affection that being with a man gives me in my life. Which means I have to go through the sex part which is not immaculate.

What I would like to remove is the sense of dirtiness, feeling used, controlling and feeling controlled that sex brings to my mind. Why again? You will say it is the programming. Can I erase it?

What I also find hard to understand is that Helios wants to give me an orgasm which is not what I asked for and makes me feel inferior/incapable/a failure to deliver. Why does he want it? Is it the same as my reasons, which are to be left in peace from my emotional demands? Why have I decided to become a rock, freezing my sexuality when men freeze their emotions but not their sexuality?

These are questions I have never been able to answer. Please help me to see with more clarity.

Thank you

Example of 'A' Type Emotional Information Deletion

One day Andrea started a session by saying that she wanted to discuss her 'tendency to dramatize,' her difficulty trusting, and how this related to her attachment strategy, which she thought might be a C+ strategy as she was starting to feel very anxious. The background for this, and what had motivated it, was this:

She had met a guy on a dating site and he was very full on in his interest in her. He said that she was just what he had been waiting for all his life. She was very flattered and taken with his attention. However, the way they were communicating, via 'Hangouts,' bothered her. (I was informed by another client that one of the appealing features of this app is that it lets you stay in contact with *all* of your contacts in one place at the same time. Very convenient if you want to have a lot of people in play at the same time.)

However, she said, she thought that there must be something wrong with her as she was having trouble trusting him. He had done nothing, she said, to cause her not to trust him. She was discounting her own negative emotions of suspicion, mistrust, and fear, by telling herself that she was being 'dramatic.' She was attributing her negative feelings to some fault in herself. But as she told me more about this interaction, I became suspicious. He was heaping her with praise and telling her that she was the woman that he had been searching for all his life and that he couldn't wait to meet her. When that could be remained unspecified due to some mystery around his work schedule.

I suspected that he was scamming her. He had made some claims that stretched the imagination: he was an Italian living in Oslo, Norway, but working in the USA. He had a PhD in psychology and a master's degree in 'satellite engineering.'

I asked the man's name and city and thought that I would Google him on the chance that he would have a webpage or some kind of presence on the internet that we could discover to check out at least some of what he was telling her. Lo and behold, there he was: 'The Phantom Scammer' on Facebook, a page created by previous victims. Of course, that did the trick, right?

Wrong. Andrea still felt guilty. It was wrong, she insisted, to make a decision about someone with whom she had formed an 'attachment relationship' based on something that someone had written about him and posted on Facebook. Never mind that what had been written on Facebook was entirely consistent with what we had supposed before ever reading the Facebook page. In her A5 mode she had formed an illusory bond. She put his needs and feelings (as he deceptively expressed them to her) ahead of her own, and she discounted my opinion due to her A6 strategy.

Because she would never dream of being intentionally deceptive to take advantage of someone else, it was hard for her to accept that others would. She felt guilty at the thought of blanking him or hurting his feelings, so she decided to give him another chance.

He assured her that he really wanted to meet her and that a good occasion to do that was to fly to London from Canada to help her celebrate her birthday that was coming up in a few weeks' time. What a guy, so self-sacrificing, so loving, so concerned with pleasing Andrea.

And oh, by the way, he didn't have any money because the gobs of money that he was due to be paid from his latest engineering work hadn't been paid yet, and so could she just advance him the money to pay for his trip? He would, of course, pay her back when his ship came in.

Andrea finally got it.

In Andrea's case, she needed the ignored emotional information that told her that something just didn't 'feel' right. Of course, the difficulty is to learn when to trust feelings and when not. A's are deleting or ignoring emotional information that lets them know they need to do something to protect themselves. They have the cognitive information, but as the strategy deepens into the higher numbers, then the factual information is distorted more and more as they move further from reality. Also, remember that the higher the numbers, the more the person's strength—cognition for A's and emotion for C's—becomes a weakness, such that the A7–8 strategies of Delusional Idealization and Externally Assembled Self represent a relatively complete distortion of the cognitive information, and on the C side, C7–8, Menacing and Paranoid, represents a relatively complete distortion of emotional information. By the time we reach AC, psychopathy, the distortions of both cognitive and emotional information are complete.

How, then, can psychopaths function so well in the real world? Because they use *balanced* information processing just as B's do. One way to think about this is that the central axis of the DMM model is going from true and accurate information processing at the top to completely distorted information processing at the bottom.

Andrea's Progress in Recovery

Andrea was moving upward near to this central axis. We can also consider Andrea's progress using Maslow's Modified Hierarchy. Her physical needs were met, however Racine had trouble with the food issue, eventually overcome. At the nurturing level, Andrea and Racine were both struggling. While they could nurture one another and had nurturing female friends, to form a nurturing relationship with a man was challenging for both. Safety and Security were fairly well accomplished, though both still struggled with fear, especially triggered by their romantic relationships but in relation to work as well. At the level of love and belonging, they were both very courageous, and while they had their struggles, both were able to take the risks that love requires. This implies that both were committed to their spiritual growth.

At the level of esteem, Andrea had won great esteem in her profession. She was consciously self-actualizing by thinking of how she could best contribute to her colleagues, her profession, and the people they served. She was also contemplating self-transcendence, reading and applying spiritual principles.

And then I got this email from Andrea:

> Dear Charley,
>
> I am reflecting on our session this morning. Thank you for helping me understand.
>
> Yes, there was sexual abuse, but it was not violent. It was a sort of desire for closeness that the abuser had because he was a sexually abused child himself and he knew only that way to have his needs met (am I correct in the way I understand this?).
>
> This makes me think the abuser came from his village to the house knowing that our parents and older siblings were not there, perhaps taking the risk of being found out with all the consequences of his wife's reaction and that of his own children (slightly older than me) to get some "affection" from two young girls like my sister and me. This was a strong drive for him who was certainly aware of the social implication of his actions but perhaps not aware of the consequences on me and my sister.
>
> Perhaps he himself never considered that he was creating two more abused human beings who may become abusers as adults and continuing his actions of abusing others.
>
> He may not even have considered that myself and my sister would feel betrayed, would lose our self-esteem, that we would believe that we <u>were</u> objects to be used. Is this *correct*?
>
> If this is the case I can confirm that I have behaved as a sex object most of my life. I have believed that the more sexual I was the more I would be loved. What came to me as a surprise is the fact that my mother and grandmother *knew* this is what happens to girls but decided to turn a blind eye and do nothing. Keep the secret making sure nobody knew. I believe in their mind it was *common and inevitable* that girls are used. Perhaps this is behind the idea I always had in mind that being born as a girl carries disgrace in society. The women carry the body that activates dirty thoughts in men. I had never considered that the men had distorted views of how to treat human beings!

> I am sure you will understand how long I have been imprisoned in these thoughts and how painful the experience has been.
> If I am lucky to have a reply from you, the other area where I wish to focus is the sense of shame that goes with the sexual abuse. This requires more thinking. Hence I will stop here. With gratitude for teaching me to care.
> Thank you
> Andrea

I did reply, and our discussion of these events and the feelings they engender continues. Notice that the opening is abstract, passive voice, very impersonal: 'Yes, there was sexual abuse, but it was not violent.' There are no people. There is gratuitous denial of a negative, 'violent.' She rationalizes the abuser's behaviour; as she goes further into it, she becomes more emotional. She speaks of being imprisoned in the past and how painful it has been. She acknowledges the shame that she has felt about it. The shame was likely there from her mother's failure to convey a sense that she is worthwhile. This made her an easy target and created fertile ground for the sexual abuse to take root. Children need attention and nurturing: touching, holding, kissing. They behave seductively in order to obtain this nurturing. Adults sometimes mistake this as behaving seductively in order to be sexually abused.

Not only that, having to 'normalize' this experience meant that it set her up for exploitation in the rest of her life. I recommended that she read Pat Carnes' *The Betrayal Bond*,[7] which describes how this process proceeds. Here is her email regarding that:

> I noted the concept of bonding with people who were hurtful and remaining loyal to them despite their betrayal and exploitation. I am interested in understanding more about this concept. This loyalty is the reason I have experienced intimate relationship difficulties in my life. This thought is mostly at the rational level. I would like to make it felt at the emotional level, which is what you usually do with me. Can we do it in our next session?

I see this as evidence that Andrea is acknowledging her loss and grief, healing her sexual abuse, her attachment wounds, and her dysfunctional relationships. Most important is her emotional engagement with this issue, her awareness of her mostly cognitive approach, and her desire to bring more emotion into it, as she is doing. I recommended that she write a letter to little Andrea expressing her feelings. Here it is:

Dear little Andrea,
When my mother went to the hospital to deliver me, I think the experience was very lonely. In my dream I was wrapped on a blanket and "parked somewhere" there was not even the presence of others in the village. I did not like the experience and I started hating you. Your presence in this world was an inconvenience, without any reason to think you had something good. I had no sympathy for this little being as a baby, as toddler, as teenager as adult.
I still hate you for existing. Your presence has ruined my life. I have treated you without any love/care. Any time there was something I was not capable of doing, I have accused you. Getting lost, fear of making mistakes, needing help are all examples. There are moments when I feel sorry for having dragged you into my life without any empathy for what you were not capable of doing. Doing was more important than being.
You were born hated by me, by my mother, by my grandmother. Why did you never rebel? I feel bad that you wanted to be cared for. Did you ask to be alive? To exist? Without you my life would have been so much easier. You were "wrong" from the beginning and I have continued to believe that I was wrong.

Notice the confusion, the incoherence, in her narrative. She is aware of this as indicated by her message to me:

Sorry Charley. This letter seems to indicate that I still hate myself. In my mind I was convinced that I had made enough progress to understand and care for the little child I have in me. On the contrary I still treat myself as an impotent kid who has never grown up! I find this refusal to grow up very sad.

I reassure her that it is alright, that this honesty, no matter how raw or unflattering, is necessary in order to move out of the first stage of the grieving process: denial. This bears fruit in our next session.

Self-hatred
Andrea begins the session by discussing her self-hatred and her goal of doing 'impossible things.' She believes that she is the most unworthy person on the planet. This belief goes all the way back to her mother learning that she was pregnant with Andrea. I reframe this as 'reverse narcissism.' She continues to reframe in a negative way, 'Oh, others are like me, but I'm the only one who makes a big deal of it.' I assure her that she doesn't make a big deal of it, rather she 'soldiers on.' I point out how well she has done in life, with her A+ strategy and the good that she has done for

others. She has trouble accepting that. I point out that this is the old script or narrative. She relates this to intergenerational trauma that she has begun to explore. She says:

> Well, I'm feeling that is what I want to do: to give myself a new script. I do want to be a better person in the sense of not blaming myself that much.
> **Blaming yourself that much for what?**
> Well, because I think I am so bad, so damaged that there is nothing good I can do.

She acknowledges her false positive affect:

> Yeah, perhaps what I am sort of aiming for is the ability to ignore the damage. To appear constantly positive, I don't know.

I remind her of the sacrifices she made to have her daughter and move to a different country to be with the father, her ex-husband, and how she has already broken out of the cycle by having a loving and very open relationship with her daughter.

> Yes and I certainly give her much more of my attention, much more of what I could give. I enjoyed her company and spending time together. I didn't treat her as a parcel to park somewhere. I have enjoyed her presence from the beginning despite the difficult marriage.
> **Yeah, and is she beautiful?**
> Yes.
> **(chuckles) that got a smile on your face. Okay so here is the trick to letting go.**
> Mm?
> **It's just information. Its information about the past, okay?**
> So can I summarise from my point of view? Having the information about the past and the generations and what probably happened to the women in my mother's line has created in me a negative belief of being and feeling worthless. Worried to have children and incapable of seeing the positive of having a child. But despite that, I have actually done my best to break free from that information from the past, to make the experience of having a child as good as possible, and actually now colleting the fruit of that beautiful, that beautiful experience.
> **Yeah, that is a really good way to put it. It takes deciding to believe something new.**
> Yeah.
> **Something that is true, yeah?**

Yeah.

And we know it's true because it helps you to deal with the situation, it is based on known facts and reality, and so it makes sense: it's logical.   Okay?

Yeah.

Okay. Another smile. I'm glad, not that I am trying to talk you out of your feelings. We are trying to change those feelings by looking at reality, okay? And the reality is, your mother could not do that. She was stuck in that old belief system, as your grandmother was, and we have talked about the reasons for that.

Yes.

And that has been a huge loss for you,

Sorry, what do you mean? What was a huge loss? The fact that my mother was stuck in old beliefs?

Yeah, the fact that your mother was incapable of loving you, the way you needed to be loved.

Yeah.

And there was something else. Your trip to your village with your sister.

Yeah?

You were really struck that all your sister wanted to do was get married and have children. Is she happy doing that?

Well, my younger sister, yes. I think my point was slightly different: that in the family I was the one that was not willing to have a family because I didn't feel comfortable to do it, and I was surprised to hear my younger sister: all she wanted was to have a family and to have children. I didn't have that instinct to want to marry. For me to have a family was to have a—to be in a prison.

You made the point: and my sister and I grew up in the same family.

mm

But you did not. Because the family your sister grew up in, she had someone in her life that you didn't have in yours. (a pause) Who was that?

Well, I think it was the husband, or the way she was accepted by the family because she was last child. I don't know.

When you say the husband?

Yeah, she found a man who was very, very caring.

What—she was born?

Oh no, no, no. Sorry. She was surrounded by the attention of the family. I mean, the first child born was a boy. A great success. Then the second came, a daughter. Okay? And then there was this interval of seven years in which I came along: another woman. And then there was the last, my younger sister two years after. But because she was the last one ... perhaps she was more cute than I was. I don't know. But she was much more err ... I felt she was much more wanted, much more liked as the last child, the cute one, or something, so ... I have seen me in the middle as the disturbing element. The one that came at the wrong moment. I have seen me as worse than the rest.

You are describing the traditional family roles of: the oldest child, the family hero, you refer to him as a great success but actually he hasn't been a great success at all, has he?

No, no.

Which often happens with family heroes. Then the second child, your older sister, she would have been in the position to be the scapegoat, to get blamed when things go wrong. You would have been the lost child, the child who is left to her own devices and that very much fits with what you described in your AAI.

[she laughs]

Oh, you are laughing.

I was laughing because I was not aware of this and yet it corresponds exactly to the way I think.

Okay, good. So it has validity. And then your younger sister, the youngest, they get to be the mascot, the baby of the family. The one that everybody loves and can do no wrong. So that's the way those family roles play out.

Yeah.

But I still haven't got the answer I am looking for.

Which is?

Which is: who did she have in her life growing up as an infant, a baby, a young child, all through her childhood, that you did not have?

Well, I suspect it could be my older brother.

No, he was there during _your_ childhood, too.

I don't know.

How about you?

Me?

Yeah?

Oh ... In what sense?

You were her older sister.

Yeah?

How did you feel toward her?

No.

No what?

I have never considered this possibility.

No, but I am asking you now, how did you feel toward her?
Well, I think I was happy. I liked her and we actually had a sort of childhood together. Yes, we did spend time together. I was, err, err … if I have a sister … I feel she is my sister, yes.

The dysfluency and not comprehending the earlier question is because her mind is engaged in reorganization, I think.

When you spent time together what was that like?
Yeah, I mean we were children together. There was two years between us and we did spend time together, yes.
Happily?
Yes.
Do you think at that time you were expressing love and acceptance to her?
I was. I think I was happy to be with her. I am sure. We have created a bond between us which has helped, yes.
Yeah, and she was happy being with you?
Mm, yes, she was. Yes, and she's … yeah.
I imagine that made a world of difference for her.
Yeah. Yes it did.
Well I think that is something very special.
mm.
What do you think?
I actually agree and I think you are right, it gave more meaning to my life, so yeah.   Yes, it did give meaning to my life, and it still does, so perhaps it … What you are saying is that it is my presence that has been beneficial to my younger sister?
Yeah.
And perhaps also beneficial to me because I had somebody that I liked who was with me.
I think that gives you a visceral understanding of what it was that you were missing, and I think you have gotten stuck in blaming and bargaining because your denial is such that you are convinced it's somehow inevitable. I think it's shifted greatly during this session, am I right?
You are right yes yes.
And that is all it is: it's letting go of that old belief and putting a new belief in which is that actually, you are loveable, you are worthwhile.
Yeah.
Yeah! Okay? Another smile, okay. A big smile this time: yeah, you are loveable, you are worthwhile, yeah. And err, you can also feel sad, as

you suffer, as you allow that loss to be processed as a loss, and I don't know how long it will take, but I don't think it will take very long, okay? Because you have been living with this loss all your life and you know, we can't change the fact of the loss but we can resolve it. We can let it move into the past instead of staying with you right now in terms of your here and now experience. You let it be in the past. You let it be resolved and you move on to acceptance, and with that acceptance comes the awareness that you are a beautiful child inside of you. You are a beautiful child. You are worthy of love, and you can give yourself that love, to fill that emptiness inside. [I point out her loving connections, especially with her daughter:] You can look at that, how the criticism she received threatened her life. Anorexia is a life threatening disease and I think she is still struggling to....

Accept herself.

Yeah. But she is well on her way, you know? Well done today.

Well, thanks to you. It is a relief to see it from a different angle. I think there is a big shift that has occurred and it has really helped me. Thank you.

You are welcome.

She bookmarks what she wants to work on next time: the belief that she needs a man in her life in order to be happy.

Rehan's Return Engagement with Us

Rehan had left the church that he had been raised in. His wife had remained a faithful church-goer. Despite having a lover for whom he cared deeply, he refused to consider leaving his wife, not that I was encouraging him to, let me quickly add. Nor was I encouraging him to break off the affair. It is not my place to tell my clients how to live their lives. That is up to them. They have to live with the consequences. He still felt a moral duty to stay and support his wife and their children, one of whom had a severe disability due in part to the effects of their strong religious beliefs at the time.

However, events eventually caught up with Rehan. Due to a shake-up at his work place, he resigned and sought employment elsewhere. This created more distress for him because he had felt very close to the team he worked with and so leaving them was a loss for him. He also had a much longer commute to work. And last but by no means least, his lover gave up on him ever leaving his wife and ended their relationship.

This was very destabilizing for Rehan, and when these events occurred he returned to therapy. We continued our work. Rehan then discovered that his former lover was living with a mutual friend to whom he had suspected she was transferring her affections. This led to a great deal of reflection on Rehan's part. He was anguished and torn. On the one hand, he missed her greatly. On the other hand, he realized that if she wanted to have children and a life with a partner, she had no choice but to break up with him and pursue a relationship with someone else.

Eventually, he decided that he wanted to contact her and let her know that he knew she was living with their mutual friend, and he wanted to wish them well. But he was afraid that it would not go well. Again, I left it to him to decide whether or not to contact her. Here is the email that I received:

> Hi Charley
> Normally, I don't ever say much between sessions and hope this isn't blurring boundaries or encroaching, but I wanted to update you as I spoke to Jasmine as I indicated I was planning to.
> She reacted really calmly and I think I managed to communicate with kindness how I felt, but also that I wanted her to be happy. It put me in mind of the definition of love as taking a risk for the betterment of someone else. I think she was genuinely moved by how I handled it. An unintended consequence (at least unconsciously) is I've felt a real spike in those limerent feelings again! I hadn't anticipated that. It's something I need to keep working on. It feels complicated, but deep down I'm glad and know it was a risk, but was something I did with good intentions consciously despite knowing she might well have reacted and said she never wanted to speak to me again!
> Thanks again for all your support and help working with me over the years. The last two weeks have been incredibly tough but I've managed with no thoughts to self-harm, turned up to work and have just about kept the panic in check. All big gains and proof of some rewiring!
> Thanks
> Rehan

Considering his A6 strategy, to share this information outside of a session was an important step for him. He apologizes for doing that. But of course, it is alright.

The definition of love that he paraphrases in the third paragraph is from Scott Peck's book, *The Road Less Travelled*.[8] Peck defines love as 'being willing to extend yourself for the spiritual growth of yourself or someone else.' Notice that in the email Rehan recast this as 'taking a risk for the betterment of someone else.' He is able to acknowledge in his description of the event his own progress: he took a risk and it paid off. But he is still focusing on helping the other person rather than himself. At the same time, he can acknowledge the limerent longing that he still feels.

In the final paragraph he gives himself credit for avoiding self-harm. He points out that he hadn't even considered it, which means that he has been successful in managing the negative emotions using other means. He also maintained emotional stability and carried on with his employment duties, whereas before he might have gone off 'sick,' too emotionally distraught to function at work. He credits himself with 'big gains' and refers to the 'emotional rewiring' that has taken place in his unconscious mind. This is actually what I refer to as 're-programming,' but hey, that is what he is referring to: the kind of deep changes in the emotional programming of the unconscious mind. For Rehan to be able to do this, and to acknowledge the loss and the pain in a constructive way, is a big deal.

He still has more work to do, but he is well on his way.

Bob's New Outlook on Life

Bob has finally ended the relationship with Tanya. I won't be surprised if she reinitiates, and he said neither will he. She has not been able to overcome the fear that she felt when he was violently angry and harming himself. After quite some time of him going around, doing chores, spending a bit of time with her sons, and having heartfelt discussions with her in which they both acknowledged how much they missed the physical intimacy and being together, and him making overtures only to be rejected, he decided to end it.

However, he has not let this bring him down. He has met someone else. Someone who is not as attractive to him, physically, as Tanya, but he likes her for who she is. Meantime, he has carried on mending his relationship with his daughters. Now he is 'knocking on the door saying "I want in."' Both daughters are responding positively, especially the oldest, Peggy. His youngest, Debbie, is still standoffish. He is not letting that put him off, he is not taking it personally. He realizes that is where she is right now, and with others as well. I got this email from Bob. It was after he had been to a performance she was in. I think it is a good indicator of the progress he has made: the new narrative:

> All in all it has been a very positive few days with Peggy and actually my mum and sister. When they arrived at the hotel yesterday I could feel all my

insecurities coming back and they hadn't actually done anything. But I used the tools I now have and was very quickly able to gather myself and we had a really nice lunch. I was in the 'here and now' through the rest of the day and evening and I really enjoyed it.

The show was amazing and my beautiful daughter was truly amazing and I was so proud, but what was new was the feeling of raw emotion watching her dance. I was really present and charged. I couldn't sleep last night because I was simply buzzing with pride and emotion of what I had just watched and felt throughout it all.

I am feeling a little flat today, work caught up with me but my resilience is so much better that it doesn't take me that long to pick myself up.

Now to engage with Debbie.

Thanks Charley.

I feel confident that Bob has turned a corner. He is attending to his business in a different way, planning ahead and enlisting help from others. He is patient and understanding with his daughters. How will this new relationship go? Well, they just met, so we shall see.

Notes

1. Gray, J., & Gray, J. (1993). *Men are from Mars, women are from Venus.* Harper Audio.
2. Pease, A., & Pease, B. (2016). *Why Men Don't Listen & Women Can't Read Maps: How to spot the differences in the way men & women think.* Hachette UK.
3. Notarius, C., & Markman, H. (1993). *We can work it out: Making sense of marital conflict.* Putnam Adult.
4. Notarius, C., & Markman, H. (1993). *We can work it out: Making sense of marital conflict.* Putnam Publishing Group.
5. Gottman, J., & Silver, N. (2015). *The seven principles for making marriage work: A practical guide from the country's foremost relationship expert.* Harmony.
6. Kandel, E. R. (2007). *In search of memory: The emergence of a new science of mind.* WW Norton & Company.
7. Carnes, P. J. (2018, August). Betrayal bond, revised: breaking free of exploitive relationships. Hci.
8. Peck, M. S. (2002). *The road less traveled: A new psychology of love, traditional values, and spiritual growth.* Simon and Schuster.

CHAPTER 10

What Could Go Wrong?

You're not a failure till you quit trying.
Zig Ziglar
Not even Jesus could save everybody.
Me

The first quote reflects the attitude of never giving up on clients. From the NLP perspective, there are no resistant clients, only non-resourceful therapists. This is in keeping with the idea that, whatever is going on with the client, if they are motivated to be there, then there is some information to be gained from what some therapists refer to as 'resistance.'

There are always going to be cases where we are not going to be successful. Hence, my own saying, which is not meant sacrilegiously but rather literally, to enable me, in those early days of learning in the treatment centre, to not fall into despair. Some people, for whatever reason, were just not going to 'get it.' Hence, my own self-protective device. And the treatment team and support staff reassured me, in those early days, that we would all have 'failures.'

When someone dies from their disease, that is a failure. When someone relapses into their addiction that can be considered a failure too. But if they remain alive and maintain their faculties, there is still hope.

C. Shults, *Attachment Centred Therapy*, Palgrave Texts in
Counselling and Psychotherapy,
https://doi.org/10.1007/978-3-031-60851-3_10

203

People leaving against medical advice (AMA) was the bane of the treatment centre. I remember one patient in particular who left AMA. He had been there less than a week, and although I was his primary counsellor, we had only met one on one on a single occasion, for about an hour. Given the threat of empty beds, when we got word that a patient was leaving AMA, we were meant to pull out all the stops in order to get them to stay. It usually didn't work.

I got word that the patient was planning to leave, so my orders were to keep him in treatment if at all possible. I tried everything that I could think of. But nothing worked. I also observed, during these attempts, that no one was ever frightened into sobriety. For this client, there was the complication of his partner who was at the end of her patience with him. Paradoxically, his fear of losing her was what he gave as his reason for leaving. But the reason that he was in danger of losing her was because of his drinking. So what was he planning to do? He was planning to leave treatment and persuade her not to leave him.

Pointing out that leaving treatment AMA was not the best way to convince her that he was serious about recovery was not persuasive. He left anyway. She was not persuaded. He resumed drinking. A week later he was dead. A single car crash. No one else involved. I wonder if that was an intentional suicide by automobile.

We have to learn to deal with our failures. Ruiz' *The Four Agreements*[1] are useful here: (1) don't take things personally; (2) always do your best; (3) never make assumptions; (4) be impeccable with your word. As with all prescriptive statements or principles of knowledge, these agreements must be correctly applied. Of course, when a client dies we feel grief. How can we not? I believe it is normal to wonder, in the blaming and bargaining phase, if we have done our best to help the client. I believe that we humans always do our best, but sometimes it's a piss poor job. In that case, is there anything that we can learn that can help us to do better next time?

There were many other failures. And out of these, one central cause was apparent: they did not follow our recommendations. Of course, that is a bit of a catch-22: don't use drugs and go to meetings. That's our recommendation. So, if you follow our recommendation, then you will remain sober. If you don't, you won't. Catch-22.[2]

Those who followed our recommendations were much more likely to be successful than those who didn't. Which brought me to another conclusion, based on observation: the point of going to a treatment centre is to convince you to do what you need to do to stay sober when you get out of the treatment centre. So, if you are willing to do what it takes to establish and maintain sobriety, then there is no need to go to the treatment centre in the first place, because nothing you can do in the treatment centre can insure sobriety and recovery when you get out. The exception is when the client is unable to do what they need in order to establish and maintain sobriety. Back to the 'always do your best' agreement, I think that we often assess that we or others have not done our best when we can look at the information cognitively and see that better could have been done. But that sort of judgement ignores the role that emotion plays in decision making and behaviour.

If we take the example of a huge failure that was a public spectacle, it was the Challenger disaster. Cognitive decision making was definitive: the launch was a no go. The temperatures were too low. The cognitive information was ignored in favour of the emotional, 'but we can't have the disappointment of another missed launch date,' and so the launch was made. The team as a whole did the best they could, and it was a piss poor job. We can learn from that mistake. Richard Feynman (winner of the Nobel prize in physics) stated the obvious: 'For a successful technology, reality must take precedence over public relations, for Nature cannot be fooled.'

With clients in private practice, the question is: do they have the discipline necessary to follow the recommendations? Of course, the techniques are much less likely to work if you haven't practised them before you need them. The perception that affirmations don't work, or Gottman's conclusion that active listening doesn't work, is based on erroneous information. They only work when you need them if you have practised them when you don't need them. So the question needs to be, not, 'Did these techniques work for you?' but rather, 'Did you work for them?' Did you put in the time and effort to learn them, to apply them, so that they work automatically and effectively whenever you need them?

A corollary is that addictive disorders are not dealt with by *not* doing the addictive behaviour, but rather by doing the things that promote recovery. What are the things that promote recovery? They are the things that you need to do to meet the unmet needs that have created the negative feelings that the addictive disorder has been medicating. And that means healing the attachment wound.

This is the connection with attachment: (1) unmet needs create negative feelings; (2) children with unmet attachment needs don't learn how to deal with their feelings effectively nor how to get their needs met; (3) addictive behaviours create good feelings that make the bad feelings go away and mask the unmet need without fulfilling it; (4) the behaviour packs a double whammy, making the bad feelings go away and creating good feelings in their stead; (5) this causes the need to increase, and so do the negative feelings that go with it; (6) simultaneously, the addictive behaviour, because it 'borrows' from other, legitimate needs without meeting those needs, becomes reinforced; (7) as the needs grow and the reward behaviour recedes in effectiveness, the addictive behaviour escalates into a disorder.

Addictive disorders arise when the unconscious mind experiences the relief from the negative feelings that the addictive disorder provides. If you are worried about life and feeling discontent, then food, heroin, and alcohol will all give you the biochemical message, 'this feels good and everything is going to be alright.'[3] If you are feeling depressed then stimulants such as cocaine and amphetamine will relieve the depression, temporarily, and you can be 'Master of the Universe.' If you feel lonely and worthless, then sex and romance can provide a temporary cure. Once the unconscious mind gets a taste of the sweet relief from negative feelings, it is going to seek it again and again. In the meantime, the unmet need grows even greater. This creates even stronger addictive urges and leads to the escalation of addictive behaviour until it becomes a disorder. At that point, the 'cure' has become worse than the disease.

It is no surprise, then, that some people are going to prefer behaviours that shorten, impair, or end their lives, when we remember the children of René Spitz' studies. When the pain of life is too great, when we lose hope, some choose death.

HONESTY, OR THE LACK THEREOF

In the 12-step programmes, one of the requirements of sobriety is what Bill Wilson, in *'The Big Book' of Alcoholics Anonymous*,[4] referred to as 'rigorous honesty.' Wilson made the claim that 'rarely' had they seen anyone fail in AA if they thoroughly follow the 12-step path. When he wrote those words, AA hadn't been around long enough for there to be that many failures. He then claimed that those who failed were unable to 'grasp and develop a manner of living that requires' this 'rigorous honesty.'

I realized early on that there was nothing I could do to prevent patients from lying to me. However, I could check out their story. There were a variety of ways that this could be done. Usually, someone came into treatment because they had been coerced into being there. Rarely did anyone wake up in the morning and think, 'Gee, I think I will go and check myself into a treatment centre today.' On the contrary, it was typically the threat of the loss of a job, a partner, or an even larger group of people who participate in an 'intervention,' typically close family and friends, who confront the person with the consequences of their behaviour in the past and the consequences that they can anticipate in the future if they don't get help. In other words, get help or else.

This coercive feature could then be used to get the patients to give permission to speak with employers, co-workers, family members, and friends. These discussions could then give us information about the problems and behaviours that had brought the patient into therapy. These discrepancies could then be queried and might lead to change. We also typically had meetings with partners, employers, and others either separately or with the patient. And then we had family week where significant others come to the treatment centre for a week where they were able to meet with other significant others in a family group. After the first couple of days spent in preparation, the patients would join us for the last three days. So, we had a number of opportunities and methods to get at the truth.

Of course, there is no guarantee that the people who are reporting on the patient are telling the truth. One of the huge advantages of the DMM-AAI and ACT are that the methodology gives us another, powerful tool to discern what is true and what is false. This comes from the discourse analysis.

People Fool Themselves

The other factor is that often people fool themselves through one of the transformations of information. That was another of Feynman's conclusions about the Challenger disaster: that the people in charge at NASA had fooled themselves. Clients have also fooled themselves. Just like NASA, they select certain information and dismiss other information in order to reconcile competing dispositional representations: different needs and beliefs. It is often the emotional, the subjective impression, that is chosen. As Simon and Garfunkel sang, we hear what we want to hear and disregard the rest. My saying for this is:

When subjective impressions are mistaken for facts,
Chaos reigns.

We see this all around us in various ways. It has been researched and books written about it. All we can do as professionals is try to learn about our own particular cognitive and emotional distortions and try to be as reality based as possible. Maybe, when we do, it will rub off on our clients.

The Hidden Agenda

Some clients are going to have hidden agendas. They have come to therapy in order to get someone off their back. They are not going to be honest with you because they don't want you to know what is going on, but they want you to *think* you know what is going on. I always suggest meeting a client's partner at least once. That way I can get a sense of who the person is that the client is describing. I can experience their personality, with the understanding that they may be presenting me with a 'false self.' Rarely do I get to meet that person. Usually the client says that their partner doesn't want to meet. However, sometimes the client is lying and telling me that their partner isn't willing to meet with us, when in fact it is the client who is using that as an excuse to not allow me to meet their partner. I have had the experience of having a partner contact me and reveal that the client had said that I did not want to meet them. So the client was playing both ends against the middle as a way to protect their secrets.

Sociopathy/Psychopathy

I use these words interchangeably. Sometimes there is a specific need to differentiate.[5] Their use is also dependent on how one defines those terms and regardless, there is a great deal of overlap. Neither are going to be honest with you. Correction: they will be honest to the extent that they use honesty to facilitate their lying. They will be charming, convincing, and the good ones will help you to feel bad for not trusting them, they will be so understanding of your doubts. In other words, they will manipulate the hell out of you, whether you are their partner or their therapist. But of course, they are not going to be in therapy with you unless they have a hidden agenda.

In training with Gottman, he advocated using pulse monitors during couple's sessions so that the couple and their therapists could tell when they were becoming 'flooded' with negative emotions. As I recall 120 beats per minute was the flooding threshold. There was an exception to this, however, he said. That exception was the sociopath. Sociopaths could remain calm in the face of marital conflict and in some cases would even become calmer, apparently finding the conflict somehow soothing.

I got to experience this with a couple that I was working with. The husband was a real estate developer. His wife stayed home and looked after the children, but now that they were grown, she was growing more discontent in the marriage. Hence, the marital therapy. I noticed that he never got upset or shouted, he stayed very calm, even condescending. And then it hit me: he was enjoying his wife's discomfort! I noticed a slight smile on his face. Next time, I asked them to wear the pulse monitors. Sure enough, hers was elevated, his was normal and actually went down at the time of his wife's upset.

In working with another couple, who did not want to do their AAIs but had done the Gottman inventory, I initially assessed him as A+ and her as C+. He was calm and reasonable while his wife was excitable and emotional. The central issue was around their adolescent child who was acting out. Mom was engaging with the child but in a conflictual way, while dad was remaining distant. But then, as I gained more information, I had an eerie realization. With dad, I could be dealing with a C5–6 strategy, which is much cooler than the C3–4, who is *intentionally* withholding support and emotional engagement from his wife. The wife, using an A3–4 strategy, can't restrain her compulsive caregiving with their child, is obsessed with everyone 'doing the right thing,' and is therefore increasingly frustrated with her husband's withdrawal and her frustration is coming out in angry outbursts, or ina's: intrusions of negative affect. If that was so and the husband was doing that intentionally, then we are indeed in the realm of sociopathy.

However, I am happy to report that the family is doing much better now. I attribute this to my wife's work with the child and the approach that I took with the parents. My approach was to focus, as always, on: (1) the identified discourse markers and correcting errors of information processing; (2) effective couple's communication techniques; (3) REBT as a way to check out their own information processing before such communications; (4) and the specific problem areas identified in the Gottman inventory. I also observed that as these techniques were applied, the wife's presentation in session became more reasonable and emotions became more manageable, and the husband became more emotionally engaging and was able to hear his wife's complaints more as a request for help with her daughter rather than a criticism of him.

Can sociopathy be identified using the AAI? That is unclear to me. According to Crittenden, psychopaths are often mis-identified as B3's! After all, they are very good at manipulating others and telling them what they want to hear.

Going Too Fast

Attachment Centred Therapy is powerful stuff. Many people experience the administration of the AAI itself as being upsetting. Others experience it as being revealing and enlightening. In fact, the final paragraph cautions that the interview might have stirred up difficult feelings and memories, and if so, then the interviewee is invited to get in touch with the interviewer for emotional support. Since the original use of the AAI was as a research instrument and then later as an assessment tool in family evaluation issues, the interviewee would normally only see the interviewer the one time, and so the invitation to get in touch if support was needed was an important caution.

In my practice, the client and I have already established a relationship, and so there is an understanding that we will be meeting again soon (usually in a week or so) and that they will have emotional support. Only once have I had an adverse reaction to the AAI itself, and that was when I did the AAI with the spouse of a client for a research project.

A few days later I got a call from her recanting everything she had said about her father in the interview. Instead, she said that he was a wonderful father, and there was an implication of blame that I had subjected her to such an unfair procedure that caused her to say such awful things. Then she revoked the permission she had previously given to use her interview in the couples study.

One might infer that she was using a C strategy.

There were a few other instances where the clients disappeared after a few sessions. I never knew for sure, but my hypothesis is that they were using an A+ strategy and the ACT process was simply too much to bear. That hasn't happened in a long time now.

I slowed down. While I want to make progress as quickly as possible, sometimes haste does make waste. Since then no one has mysteriously disappeared. That means paying careful attention to the ZPD. Too fast is overwhelming, too slow is boring.

Learn from your mistakes.

Going Too Slow

And now for the other side of the coin. Sometimes therapy fails because we can't go fast enough. One case in particular where this happened was with a client who was in a very cognitively oriented line of work. He had a rigid belief about 'right' and 'wrong.' This led to conflict with his superiors and those he managed. He couldn't seem to understand why he was being cautioned for doing 'the right thing' by giving a hard time to someone who had done 'the wrong thing.'

He was also engaging in the same kind of behaviour with his family. I expressed my concern that his employer was not going to tolerate his behaviour much longer. He responded from the rather imperious position that he was doing the right thing and so why should they fire him?

Sure enough, he cancelled his next appointment because he had been fired. And even though I reached out and tried to persuade him to carry on therapy for the benefit of him and his family, he did not reply.

Sometimes events overtake us before we are prepared to deal with them successfully.

Provocative Partners

Another difficulty is partners who are not supportive. Unsurprisingly, some of the most provocative partners have been therapists in training or newly minted. I suppose that it provides proof for the adage that a little knowledge can be a dangerous thing. The other factor is that these new therapists had always been trained in a singular technique. They then—according to my clients who have been blessed with a partner who is learning to be a therapist—use this technique as a cudgel to bludgeon the client into submission without considering that their technique might not be the best one to use in this situation. Regardless, the clients already had a therapist: me. What they needed was a partner.

Not all provocative partners are therapists in training. Another, Gregory's partner, for example, was in another helping profession—the sort of profession that often has the role of advising others to get help. Over the years that we worked together, Gregory's story was consistent that his partner was doing things intentionally to wind him up. On occasion, she would admit this to him.

This raises a moral, ethical, and perhaps legal dilemma: what does one do when one suspects that this client would be better off without this person for a partner? I think the answer is obvious: it is not my place to make a decision or even suggest a decision for my client. Why is it not? It is not for a moral, ethical, or legal reason, although those are all significant considerations. It is practical. The client has to live with the consequences of their decision. And I can't know the 'truth' of the situation. All I can know is the representation that the client has given me. My job is to help them explore their options and then support them whichever way they choose to go.

What I have experienced is numerous clients who have been in a relationship with someone who was not helpful to them. And then, *voila*, when they left that relationship, they fairly quickly found someone with whom to be in a healthy and happy relationship. This has happened fairly consistently with clients who do decide, after a period of work, to move on. But not always, as Andrea's story shows.

In fact, that was one of the factors that I noted early on to conclude that ACT was a more effective method of working than I had used in the past. The most striking I will call Linda. She was in a relationship with a man who, by her report, treated her badly. Of course, getting such a report is not unusual, and even working with couples, the biggest challenge is to get them to stop blaming each other for the problems, and instead to focus on what they can do to make the relationship better. In this case, Linda made the decision, after a few years of work, to leave her current partner. It was not long until she had met someone with whom she reported being very happy. She ended therapy, and I have not heard from her since. And, there were two more with similar stories and outcomes in those early days.

The other side of the coin is the partner who comes to therapy in support of the client. What I have experienced with several clients who have rather high numbered strategies, the partners who come to support them have been B's, in my opinion. They have been helpful, understanding, and without blame or complaining. Their attitude has been, 'What can I do to help?'

There have not been that many of them. However, the consistency has been noticeable.

SECONDARY GAIN AND NO DESIRE TO CHANGE

Q—How many therapists does it take to change a light bulb?
A—Only one, but the light bulb has to really want to change.

Forgive the old joke, but it is a way to introduce the idea that, sometimes, clients just really don't want to change. People sometimes come to therapy for reasons other than to change themselves. Back to the lack of honesty, in some cases, clients have come to therapy (or the treatment centre) in order to get their partner, or parents, employer, the legal system, or some other third party off their backs. Of course, anyone who has done couple's therapy for any length of time will have experienced the phenomenon of 'I'm here to get help fixing my partner.' The most challenging aspect of couple's therapy early on is to get each person to look at themselves and how they can change rather than to try to get their partner to change.

MASKING TRAUMA, LOSS, OR DISABILITY

This describes situations where the client is exhibiting insecure attachment but is unable to correctly attribute this condition to early developmental deficits due to accompanying or subsequent trauma, loss, or disability. This masks the original contributing factor of insensitive, unresponsive parenting with an obvious and undeniable condition or circumstance that is going to have a developmental impact and does contribute to the attachment insecurity.

Medical conditions, parental loss through death or divorce, or other ACEs (adverse childhood experiences) are painfully obvious to the client and are undeniable. Some clients who are well defended are unwilling to look beyond these ACEs to the original and underlying attachment relationships. Of course, we can point this out to the clients, but they are not necessarily going to buy into that theory. I have had a few clients with whom I believe this to have been the case, and the intervening ACE has impeded progress.

I don't assume that an ACE is going to have this effect. They usually don't. I follow the evidence. I have had at least one client who did have, so far as I could tell, a secure relationship with her parents up until age 3 when her mom became psychotic and her father abusive towards her mother. These ACEs totally upset the secure setting in which she had spent her first three years and she developed an A3/4 strategy in subsequent years. The evidence that I have of the validity of this hypothesis is, first, that we got confirming evidence of this from her unconscious mind in the TLT® process, and second, that couple's therapy for her and her husband based on this hypothesis was successful since they went from being on the brink of divorce to being happily married once again.

What can we take from these observations? Follow the evidence. In the cases that were not successful, the clients were unwilling to even consider the evidence that insecure attachment was preceding the ACEs or developed concurrently. All was attributed to the ACE despite the evidence to the contrary. This comingled with the C4 strategy that maintained victimhood. From this stance, which in previous contexts elicited care-giving, any attempts at changing their narrative were seen as threats, not aids.

DEFENSIVENESS

Last but not least, there is just good, old-fashioned, defensiveness. The key is to identify the defences being used, to understand the purpose that is being served, and to develop alternatives. Denial is the big one. We sometimes choose to deny unpleasant aspects of reality.

NOTES

1. Ruiz, D. M., & Mills, J. (2011). *The Four Agreements (Illustrated Edition): A Practical Guide to Personal Freedom (Four-color Illustrated Ed.)*. Hay House, Inc.
2. Heller, J. (1999). *Catch-22: a novel* (Vol. 4). Simon and Schuster.
3. Milkman, H. B., & Sunderwirth, S. G. (2009). *Craving for ecstasy and natural highs: A positive approach to mood alteration*. Sage.
4. Alcoholics Anonymous by Bill Wilson, one of the two founders of AA.
5. Pemment, J. (2013). Psychopathy versus sociopathy: Why the distinction has become crucial. *Aggression and Violent Behavior, 18*(5), 458–461.

CHAPTER 11

An Afterword and Acknowledgements

I hope this book will be of some use to you. One interesting facet that is exemplary of the ongoing recursive character of this method came about serendipitously, as much else has, during the final phase of preparing for publication. As a part of that process, I sent my clients the sections of the book that applied to them to make sure that they were still okay with giving me permission to use their stories and also to allow for any corrections that they wanted to make. This resulted in spontaneous expressions of their own progress, their own shock of recognition in seeing their journey through my description of my experience with them. This has resulted, I hope, in renewed hope, and in a new awareness of the progress they have made in overcoming their insecure attachments.

It also suggests to me that further exploration of this reflective function holds further promise of 'extension and refinement' (to quote, once again, Bowlby and Ainsworth) of these techniques. It also suggests to me that perhaps we have come full circle, back to Carl Rogers' proposition[1] that reflection of the client's experience, without judgement, is the correct approach. But whereas Rogers' approach was, in my opinion, entirely too subjective to be successful, combining the Rogerian aspects of unconditional positive regard, empathy, and congruence, with the methodology of ACT, is both accepting and collaborative in striving for self-actualization *a la* Maslow, his fellow humanist. I hope that this accepting, collaborative,

© The Author(s), under exclusive license to Springer Nature Switzerland AG 2024
C. Shults, *Attachment Centred Therapy*, Palgrave Texts in Counselling and Psychotherapy,
https://doi.org/10.1007/978-3-031-60851-3_11

non-judgemental approach has come through in the previous chapters. I distinguish here between judging the person versus having an opinion about the efficacy of the behaviour.

ACKNOWLEDGEMENTS

There are many people to whom I owe gratitude for this book being published. I have no doubt that there are some whom I will inadvertently overlook, for which (like any good A+ strategist) I will apologize in advance! There are many others that I will include in reference to the organizations in which we jointly served. This is intentional due to limitations of time and space and also to provide some degree of cover for the first category! Those that I will name here are the ones who stand out in my mind, both for the length of our association and for the depth of our exploration.

I begin with the most important, the most pervasive, and that is my wife, Louise, or Dr Louise Atkin in her capacity as a child and adolescent psychiatrist and therapist. We met at the International Association for the Study of Attachment (IASA) conference in Frankfurt, Germany, in September, 2012. Given that she works primarily with children and young adults on attachment issues and I work with adults and couples, it was, one might say, a marriage made in heaven. Together we have explored ideas, techniques, and possibilities with regard to both our personal and professional evolution in attachment. We practise what we preach, if you will forgive another religious allusion. Our life together is the living embodiment of what I am presenting here. More important for the thesis of this book, Louise began to apply the ideas and methods of Attachment Centred Therapy (ACT) with her clients, or patients in the medical setting, and had immediate success, as I did when I first began to explore the concept. She has also been very patient as I have devoted significant time to getting this book done. It's only taken me 20+ years!

Next is Dr Arlene Vetere, my supervisor, my mentor, my friend. Arlene, a highly accomplished practitioner, author, and clinician, encouraged me to submit this book to Palgrave for publication in their Palgrave Texts in Counselling and Psychotherapy series. It had never occurred to me to have the temerity to write a book for other professionals to use. Arlene encouraged me to do so, and with her guidance and that of her colleague, who is next in this list, the book has been shepherded into what it is now. Arlene has been my support throughout the process. It was she who first recognized the resemblance of Attachment Narrative Therapy (ANT) to Attachment Centred Therapy.

My intent initially was to write a book that might be of interest to anyone, both therapists, their clients, and do-it-yourselfers who wanted guidance in their own journey of recovery. It also addressed a number of societal issues, including cosmology. It was Arlene who suggested that I pare it down to a focused book for therapists. I am glad she did.

Her co-author and co-creator of ANT, Dr Rudi Dallos, then took over the task of actually editing the book into the final version to be submitted to Palgrave. Rudi has been a good editor. He has advised, questioned, and cajoled me into making changes that make the book more succinct, more evidence-based, more directly relevant to the subject that it purports to treat. I can feel his excitement at interacting with two approaches, ANT and ACT, that have so much in common. To have two such accomplished scholars and clinicians assisting me has been a great blessing. I am very thankful for their generosity and giving spirit. And thank you to the folks at Palgrave/Springer for agreeing to publish this book and for bringing it to fruition: Liam Inscoe-Jones, Raghupathy Kalynaraman, and Linda Irudhayaraj.

Of course, as you have discovered in reading this book, Dr Paticia Crittenden and the Dynamic Maturational Model of Attachment (DMM) plays a leading role. It was Pat who recommended Arlene when I was looking for a supervisor knowledgeable about attachment. It was Pat who explained to me the difference between the mainstream model of attachment in the USA, the Berkely or ABC+D model, and the DMM, and why the research articles I was reading were not lending clarity to my understanding of attachment, but rather confusion, because it did not make sense. It was her elucidation of the DMM that has led me to my understanding of attachment today. And if I've got any of it wrong, then that is my error, not hers. I am amazed at what she has done. It is tempting to say 'single-handedly,' but that is not quite right. She has had many colleagues along the way who have helped her in developing and promoting her model. Many of them have been important to me in my development as well. Andrea Landini is her primary collaborator. He is the co-author of their book, *Assessing Adult Attachment*,[2] and was her co-trainer as well in our training course. There are many others, of course. And this is where I restrain myself, because if I name one, or a few, I will miss out others.

Pat had the courage to break out on her own. To look at new data with new eyes. To actualize her belief that in the discrepancies lies the new learning. It is this spirit of intellectual enquiry that has led to her expansion of the original Ainsworth categories into the current DMM model. She has indeed been true to the vision of Bowlby and Ainsworth that their model would be 'refined and extended,' to use their words. She has had the courage to endure shunning by her peers in the attachment establishment because she could not agree that it was safety that organized attachment, that the best we could do with new patterns of attachment was to label them 'disorganized,' or that attachment was 'transmitted' from mother to child in some mysterious way. Although I was not present in those early days, I was early enough to be a founding member of the International Association for the Study of Attachment in 2007.

I also have great gratitude for another mentor, teacher, and colleague, Dr Patrick Carnes. I met Pat Carnes at a South-Eastern Conference on Alcohol and Drugs in Atlanta, Georgia. We had a long association before I came to the UK. I was active in the International Institute of Trauma and Addiction Professionals and the National Council on Sexual Addiction and Compulsivity (now the Society for the Advancement of Sexual Health) and served on the boards of both those organizations. It was my years of service on those boards and the commensurate rewards that led me to assiduously resist the temptations to serve on the IASA board!

Pat Carnes, like Pat Crittenden, has written many books, trained many therapists, and broken new ground in their fields. I have found it very exciting to be in on the cutting edge of development in both the addiction and trauma and the attachment field. It was with Pat Carnes that I first discussed my ideas regarding addiction, attachment, and trauma that are presented in this book.

Special thanks, too, to my very first supervisors, Robbin McInturff and Jim Cotton at Adult and Child Development Professionals in Birmingham, Alabama. Robbin was my official supervisor and Jim was an unofficial supervisor. During that time Robbin was voted Supervisor of the Year by the American Counselling Association. I had nothing to do with her winning that honour. Again, I feel deeply fortunate to have had such an accomplished supervisor, colleague, and mentor. Jim and Robbin were like mom and dad guiding my first steps as a therapist. Another supervisor from that period was Dr Don Brown. I was a member of Don's systemic family therapists supervision group until I left to come to England. Don was instrumental in getting licensure for marriage and family therapists in Alabama and an active member of the American Association for Marriage and Family Therapists.

Thanks to Parkside Lodge, Warrior, Alabama, for giving me my first job as a counsellor and for the training they gave me. Thanks to Morris Hamilton, the executive director who hired me and who ran the treatment centre to make it one of the best. Thanks to John Nicolini, the treatment director and later my colleague at Alabama Therapy Associates, for his guidance of the treatment team. To Randy Walton, the family week director, who gave me and guided me in my first experience of working with families and then trusted me to fill in for him as family week facilitator. Also to Dr Larry Bannon, our staff psychologist, who provided us with psychological insight into our patients and guided us in using it in our work with them.

I also want to acknowledge the contribution of my late wife, Dr Nanci Turner-Shults. She had achieved her dream of becoming a professor at the University of Alabama when she was tragically struck with illness that quickly led to her death. It was she who suggested to me that I become a counsellor. She stood by me during my active addiction disorder and into recovery. She helped me get my start in counselling with my first job at the treatment centre. She introduced me to the idea of Bowlby's attachment theory, and the rudimentary A, B, and C attachment strategies.

Thanks to John Kitchens, my friend, colleague, and professor, at Birmingham-Southern College, and for many years and adventures afterwards, for introducing me to Ellis' Rational Emotive Behaviour therapy and Abraham Maslow's hierarchy of needs. Thanks to Mary Lucas Powell, also a friend from BSC, who read the manuscript and gave me advice and encouragement.

There are many others, of course, and when I think of the many friends, colleagues, and teachers over the years, I smile with gladness and tears come into my eyes. So please forgive me for not naming you all.

I also want to thank my parents. They did the best they could, even though in many ways it was a piss-poor job. As with most parents, they wanted better lives for their children than they had themselves. They succeeded in that in spite of having to struggle with their own demons: their own abuse, their own addictions, their own shame. And even though they were not always impeccable with their word, they gave me a commitment to some kind of integrity, where one must account to oneself for one's actions in life. They instilled an ethic of being kind to others, of looking down on no one, because there but for circumstance go I, and of being unimpressed by material wealth because there but for circumstance go any of us. Whatever else, they helped me to realize that our circumstances in life determine who we are, what we believe, and how we treat others. And most of all, in the realm of trauma and addiction, they gave me a lot of good material to work with!

And finally, I am deeply grateful to my clients who have taught me so much over the years. I am especially grateful for those who have allowed me to share their stories with you. Their willingness to be vulnerable, their commitment, their dedication to making their lives, and the lives of others better have been steadfast. To trust me to share their journey with them has been an honour. Remember:

> *It takes courage to grow up*
> *And become*
> *Who you really are.*
>
> e.e. cummings

NOTES

1. Rogers, C. (2012). *Client centered therapy* (new ed). Hachette UK.
2. Crittenden, P. M., & Landini, A. (2011). *Assessing adult attachment: A dynamic-maturational approach to discourse analysis.* WW Norton & Company.

Appendix A: Refinement and Extension

Bowlby and Ainsworth anticipated 'refinement and extension' of the ABC model. Both subsequent models—the Berkeley or ABC+D and the DMM—more or less agree on the B1–5 and A1–2 and C1–2 classifications, as classifications, but not on others. They do not agree on whose AAIs would be classified in which category.

B strategists are unlikely to appear in therapy unless it is in support of someone else. Here are the B categories, for comparison:

Dynamic Maturational Model (DMM)	Berkeley Model (ABC+D)
B	B= F (Free, Secure-autonomous)
B1. Distanced from past	F1. Some setting aside of attachment
	F1a. Re-evaluation and redirection of personal life as the successor to a harsh childhood
	F1b. Limited involvement with attachment
B2. Accepting	F2. Somewhat dismissing or restricting of attachment
B3. Comfortably balanced	F3. Prototypically secure/autonomous
	F3a. Continuous secure
	F3b. Earned secure
B4. Sentimental	F4. Strong expressed valuing of relationship, accompanied by some manifestations of preoccupation with attachment figures, or past trauma
	F4a. Sentimental regarding attachment

(continued)

© The Author(s), under exclusive license to Springer Nature
Switzerland AG 2024
C. Shults, *Attachment Centred Therapy*, Palgrave Texts in
Counselling and Psychotherapy,
https://doi.org/10.1007/978-3-031-60851-3

(continued)

	F4b. Mild preoccupation with unfortunate parenting experiences
B5. Complaining acceptance	F5. Somewhat resentful/conflicted while accepting of continuing involvement
BO. Balanced Other (meet the general criteria for a balanced strategy, but do not fit the criteria for any of the particular Type B strategies)	

As you can see from the above comparison, there isn't a great deal of difference between the two. They agree that the B1–2 categories are more distanced, or cooler, regarding attachment relationships, that the B3 is the attachment 'gold standard,' and that the B4–5 are more emotionally engaged with attachment relationships. As you can also see, there are a plethora of subcategories within the F strategy in the Berkeley model. Why there need to be so many at this level is a bit hard to understand. Since people using a B strategy generally have no difficulty with attachment relationships, this seems to be an academic exercise having little clinical relevance.

Here are the A categories:

Dynamic Maturational Model (DMM)	Berkeley Model (ABC+D)
A	A= Ds (Dismissing of attachment)
A1. Idealizing	Ds1. Dismissing of attachment
A2. Distancing	Ds2. Devaluing of attachment
A3. Compulsive Caregiving	Ds3. Restricted in feeling
	Ds3a. Prototypic
	DS3b. Absent, inconsistent, or contradicted indices of valuing attachment at an emotional level
A4. Compulsive Compliance/Performance	Ds4. Cut-off from source of fear of death of the child
A5. Compulsive Promiscuity	
A6. Compulsive Self-reliance	
A7. Delusional Idealization	
A8. Externally Assembled Self	

In my opinion the description of the Ds (A) category as 'Dismissing of Attachment' is wrong. A's are not at all dismissing of *attachment*. What they dismiss are their negative feelings and their own needs in order to form and maintain attachment relationships.

Here are the C categories:

Dynamic Maturational Model (DMM)	Berkeley Model (ABC+D)
C	C= E (Entangled, Preoccupied with or by early attachment or attachment-related experiences)
C1. Threateningly angry	E1. Passive
C2. Disarmingly desirous of comfort	E2. Angry/conflicted
C3. Aggressive anger	E3. Fearfully preoccupied by traumatic events
	E3a. Confused fearful and overwhelmed by traumatic/frightening experiences
	E3b. Distressing loss of memory in apparent relation to traumatic experiences
C4. Feigned helpless	
C5. Punitive	
C6. Seductive	
C7. Menacing	
C8. Paranoid	

Appendix B: REBT Worksheet

ACTIVATING EVENT (the facts of what happened)
BELIEF (what you tell yourself about the Activating Event)
CONSEQUENCE (feelings and behaviours that you don't like)
THREE QUESTIONS:

1. Does my belief help me in the long run?
2. Is my belief consistent with known facts and reality?
3. Is my belief logical?

If 'no' to *any* of these, then the belief is IRRATIONAL: go on to D.
DISPUTE THE IRRATIONAL BELIEF (tell yourself something new and healthy that is rational and you can answer 'yes' to the three questions above)
EFFECTIVE NEW EMOTIONS (new feelings and behaviours that help)

C. Shults, *Attachment Centred Therapy*, Palgrave Texts in Counselling and Psychotherapy, https://doi.org/10.1007/978-3-031-60851-3

INDEX[1]

[1] Note: Page numbers followed by 'n' refer to notes.